BACKPACK & BEYOND

DISCOVERING THE KEYS TO THE KINGDOM

*Jasnyne
I love you!*

STACY DODD
Author, Speaker, Certified Interventionist

Stacy Dodd

Dodd Publications

BACKPACK AND BEYOND. Copyright © 2024 by Stacy Dodd Dodd Publications. All rights reserved. Printed in the United States of America. No part of this book may be used or reproduced in any manner whatsoever without written permission except in the case of brief quotations embodied in critical articles and reviews. For information, contact Stacy Dodd, 1709 Linden Dr., Nesbit, Mississippi 38651

FIRST EDITION

Artwork Credits:

Cover Design: Trish Toomey, Masena Media Productions, LLC.,

Artwork illustration : Angus.YW, Ирина Батюк, Getty Signature Images

Page 11: Artwork Concept Design: Trish Toomey; Artwork Illustration: norbertsobolewski, JoyImage

Page 51: Artwork Concept Design: Trish Toomey; Artwork Illustration: Dzianis Vasilyeu, microvone

Page 82: Artwork Concept Design: Trish Toomey, Artwork Elements: AI Chat-GPT

Photo credits unless otherwise noted: Stacy Dodd

Edited by Trish Toomey, Masena Media Productions, LLC.

Hard Cover ISBN: 978-1-7363368-3-0

Paperback ISBN: 978-1-7363368-5-4

Masena Media Productions, LLC.

Foreword

Stacy Dodd is one of those people who cannot simply be a stranger in the room. From the moment I met him in a Celebrate Recovery meeting at our church, I knew there was something different about him. Many of the people who came to our Recovery sessions were dealing with problems that seemed insurmountable. Some were just going through the motions of recovery to check a box with a parole officer or angry spouse. And some, like Stacy, were communicating hope.

When you meet some people, they may shake your hand, but their eyes are elsewhere, and so is their mind. You are sure that before they let go of your hand, they've forgotten your name. But it was never that way with Stacy. In that first meeting, he'd walked around the room meeting people, asking about their lives, their struggles, their day. It was like playing twenty questions. Every contact he made was intentional. Every person was looked full in the face and square in the eye. I wondered briefly if he was running for public office, and was positive he'd already forgotten my name. Instead, when it came time for a small group breakout session where we could pray together, Stacy led the men in prayer, and prayed for every man in that room by name, even naming issues they were dealing with, relatives with health issues, the works. He'd not forgotten my name, or the name of anyone in there.

Stacy's backstory is riveting. At his lowest, he was

homeless, living out of a backpack and running through the woods outside Joplin Missouri, with nobody left that he could turn to. He'd burned all the bridges, and there wasn't a door left that could open to him. He prayed for help at that low point, turning to the only one left who had never rejected him - though he'd never really called out to him before. God had an answer for Stacy... he got arrested. Seems a bum response to a heartfelt cry for help, but God is amazing at doing the impossible with the unexpected.

From that low pit, God took Stacy on a rocket ride, to a place of respect, authority, and leadership. Stacy is now a multi-published author and speaker, an effective evangelist, and a community leader. He is a Certified Addiction Interventionist, a Director at the city's Chamber of Commerce, and a State Representative for Celebrate Recovery. It's been a joy watching him fill new exciting roles each year, expanding his horizons. It's been a joy, but it's not been a big surprise.

First, because that direct manner of his, the genuine warmth and respect he showed to everyone he met, was powerful. From the mayor of a city to a down-and-out convict or a homeless addict on the street, Stacy treats them all the same. And that doesn't happen without lasting change in the lives he touches. And second, because it's not been him doing all this - it's been God doing it all through a yielded vessel. I've heard Stacy say before that if God could use a talking donkey, then he can use me.

This is true of you, too. God can use anyone to accomplish

Foreword

great things. Even you. The book in your hands is Stacy's powerful attempt to pass on some of the life lessons he's learned in the trenches - the Kingdom Keys. These keys are ideas and means Stacy used to open the doors to Leadership, Community, Recovery, Ministry, and Mentorship. At that low point, all these doors were shut to him. The locked door is a constant symbol to a homeless person of the world shutting you out - of the limitations put on you by a society that has rejected you. But Stacy didn't stay down there, and if you're there, you don't have to stay there, either.

Use the keys Stacy describes, and the assistance God provides, to open those doors and come into the light, and find out what an amazing future God has for you.

~ Chris Solas, Author

Editor's Note

A simple lock and key.

These are everyday household things: the key to a car, a door, a safe. When these keys were first made, we guarded them as precious things and always kept them close. We knew without these keys, we couldn't access important places or our most secret treasured items.

As time passes and we gather more keys, old ones are discarded or put into that junk drawer we all have. Eventually, we forget what these keys were supposed to unlock.

Until one day, we find that old locked suitcase or file cabinet. We go to our stash of keys and try to find the one that unlocks the door to the "hidden treasure." We keep trying every key, but none of them fit. Just as we are about to give up, we find the right key, and a wave of triumph and satisfaction washes over us.

Not just any key would fit into a specific lock. The key we needed had unique properties that no other key had. Specific grooves or notches made that one key the perfect fit.

But, a *master key* - that changes everything. A master key opens all the locks, no matter what they are. In the spiritual sense, a master key represents the transformative power of faith. It gives full access to hidden places and items others may have lost or discarded, just as faith can open up new perspectives and opportunities in our lives.

People who suffer from addiction are like a hidden treasure. They are the ones who have deep secrets inside that are hidden away from others. You may find a stray key that opens one area of their life, but you'll only scratch the surface without full access.

Master keys are needed to open these access points into the lives of people who are hurting, struggling, and trying their best to pull it together. Multiple master keys fit in every lock. Using these keys, we can unlock some of the greatest treasures in the people that God loves.

So, the question is, how does someone get the Master Keys? The answer is easy: they are only given by the Master. Once you've submitted your life to Jesus Christ, He leads us to His marvelous goal for our lives. Along the way, we'll find Master Keys that He has for us to open doors into other people's lives, unlocking those hidden treasures so that they can obtain their Master Keys. This continues until God is ready for us to come home with Him.

As you read further into Stacy's book, you will discover these Access Points and Master Keys that God has given him. He has been blessed to be able to use each one of these to unlock the hidden treasures that God has put in his path.

What's stopping you from finding your Master Keys? God has them ready for you; all you need to do is accept His Eternal

Gift of Salvation to open the first door.

~ Trish Toomey, Editor

Introduction

I never dreamed in a million years that I would write a book, much less a fourth one. My first book, "Backpack to the 'Burbs," my life story, and my second book, "Outcast to Executive," have been distributed in recovery centers, jails, prisons, homeless shelters, schools, and on the streets across the USA for many years now.

Since the release of my books, the windows of Heaven have opened wide. So many things have happened. In each immense blessing, God has repeatedly proven His faithfulness and commitment to honoring His word and promises.

During the first half of my life, I lived without God. Since my life transformation at age 33, I've discovered a life I never knew existed. I found this life as I began studying and applying the scriptures in my life. As I learned to allow God to lead me through the power of His Holy Spirit, I started experiencing the promises coming to life. It has been more overwhelming as each day passes.

My life has been a true story of a journey to the bottom of the pit and into the Kingdom of Heaven on earth. God laid it on my heart to write this new book, which describes ways to access the Kingdom in detail. I share what I've come to call the Keys to the Kingdom.

Today, I've discovered the treasure of helping those overcoming addiction, alcoholism, and mental health issues, as well as those leaders stepping into executive-level leadership positions, learn how to activate the promises in God's word to reach their full potential and discover the beautiful experience of living their best life.

I'm so incredibly excited to share critical insights and principles that God has repeatedly proven to me as absolute truths.

I spent my early years as a latch-key kid raised by a single mother. My teenage and early adult life was spent as a homeless addict. I finally hit rock bottom, unsure why I was alive, then discovered the most extraordinary gift known to mankind at the most unlikely place. I began a career in ministry and non-profit leadership and eventually landed an incredible job in the addiction recovery field, becoming a respected community and executive-level professional.

Spiritual Leadership is the power to change the atmosphere through one's presence, the unconscious influence that makes Christ and spiritual things real to others. When our souls are healthy, we change the environment; the environment doesn't change us.

"For we are God's handiwork, created in Christ Jesus to do good works, which God prepared in advance for us to do."

Ephesians 2:10 NCV

During the past two decades of my personal and professional life, God has revealed that life viewed from a Kingdom perspective leads to a beautiful existence. This perspective also leads to the impact and long-term outcomes we bring into the lives of those we love and lead.

Everything I am and all I do each day is because of Jesus. The Keys to the Kingdom illustrated in the book are the access points and platforms God has revealed to me that grant access to His kingdom.

Experiencing God's kingdom in this lifetime is the greatest gift imaginable. I'm eternally grateful to God for revealing where the true treasure lies.

The organizations, ministries, and communities in which we live and serve are our responsibilities. The Kingdom perspective is life viewed per the spiritual principles and truths that have always stood the test of time.

The art of being led by God is a learned skill. This skill is developed over time as we test and prove that God is faithful and His promises come to pass when we follow His instructions.

"When all else fails, read the instructions."

In life, God has given us His instructions.

Introduction

I'm so excited to share the incredible Key Principles of spirituality, recovery, leadership, community, ministry, and mentorship that, if put into practice, will lead to the most beautiful, fulfilling, and productive life.

"Whoever believes in Me, as the Scripture has said, 'Out of his heart will flow rivers of living water."

John 7:38 Amplified Bible

Introduction

We are doorways to the Kingdom. As spirit-filled believers, we should radiate God's love and joy wherever we go. We should be the vessels that God uses to invite others in.

ACCESS POINTS AND MASTER KEYS

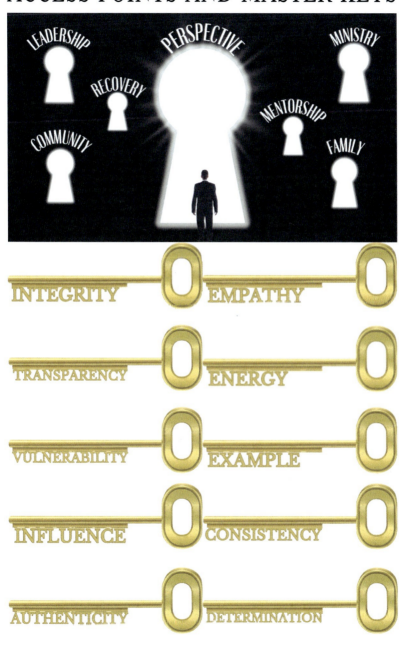

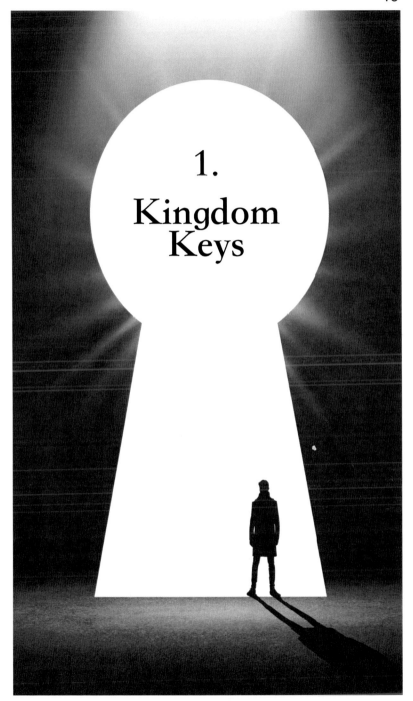

Keys are defined as gaining or preventing entrance, possession, or control.

We always keep our keys with us in case we need them.

The Keys to the Kingdom described in this book are the key platforms, or access points, and principles that give us access to the Kingdom of God on this earth in this life.

The Access Points are Leadership, Community, Recovery, Perspective, Ministry, Mentorship, and Family.

The Master Keys to accessing the hearts and minds of those I encounter are empathy, integrity, vulnerability, example, determination, transparency, influence, authenticity, energy, consistency, and many others. When we love and lead as God instructs and as the Spirit leads, we will witness miracles daily.

As God leads us intentionally to the people, places, and things he has designed for us, we will be on the supernatural adventure of a lifetime every day.

When we follow Him wholeheartedly, each encounter with human beings is a divine appointment. My life has proven that He has very specific assignments for each of us. He needs us to do what He has called and assigned us.

The Helper

In this life, we will all encounter the good and the bad. We will be forced to endure many challenges. Some will be our fault, and some will not.

The GREAT NEWS is that we don't have to depend solely on our strength, wisdom, and resources to succeed.

No force in the Universe can deliver what the Holy Spirit can deliver. No force in the Universe has the ability or power to deliver what the Holy Spirit can and does deliver.

No book, organization, group, leader, church, pastor, looks, money, power, church, school, university, or even degree can deliver what the Holy Spirit delivers.

Only the Holy Spirit of the living God can deliver the PASSION, FIRE, ENERGY, LOVE, CONVICTION, DISCERNMENT, JOY, PEACE, KINDNESS, CONTENTMENT, GENTLENESS, and GUIDANCE that is from God.

The Holy Spirit is the empowerment of God to help you do what you cannot do.

The Helper does just that. The Holy Spirit helps us do what we could never do alone, as the scriptures assure us.

"But the Comforter (Counselor, Helper, Intercessor, Advocate, Strengthener, Standby), the Holy Spirit, Whom the Father will send in My name [in My place, to represent Me and act on My behalf], He will teach you all things. And He will cause you to recall (will remind you of, bring to your remembrance) everything I have told you."

John 14:26 Amplified

When we give our lives to Christ, the Holy Spirit permanently resides in the believer's body. From that moment on, God works in and through us on this earth.

One of the most mind-blowing revelations is that when the Holy Spirit takes residence in our bodies, we instantly become Mobile Vessels of His love.

He leads and guides us intentionally and precisely to people, places, and things to help us accomplish the specific assignments He's designed and prepared us to do in advance.

We must explore the spirit-filled life, for it is by the power of the Spirit, not our power, that we continue Jesus's work in this world.

As we grow and work through the Sanctification process, our goal is to become more like Christ and lead others to him through our words and example.

> Yield myself to God to be used to bring this Good News to others, both by my example and my words. *Celebrate Recovery, Principle 8*

"Little children, let us stop just saying we love people; let us really love them, and show it by our actions."

1 John 3:18 TLB

Believer vs. Follower

I've discovered significant, visible, and noticeable differences between a Believer in Christ and a Follower of Christ. I've encountered and still encounter daily those who claim to be Christians but do not follow Him in their actions.

Romans tell us that if you confess with your mouth that Jesus is Lord and believe in your heart that God raised Him from the dead, you will be saved. ***Romans 10:9 NIV***

If we believe Jesus was born of a virgin, lived a sinless life, died on the cross for our sins, and rose again, and we put our faith in Him, we will be saved. Our salvation is secure. No one can take that from us. The world didn't give it, and the world can't take it away. Our enemies, friends, families, society, the rich, the powerful, politicians, and not even pastors can take that or disqualify us from our free gift of Salvation.

The promises in God's word must be activated. One can read the Bible daily for the rest of their lives and not obtain the promises. One can recite the entire Bible and still not experience the riches of God's promises coming to pass in this life.

As with any endeavor in life, "Action Activates." For years, I've encountered men and women who have obvious gifts and strong callings but absolutely refuse to engage in the mission. I've witnessed them make excuses, divert attention, blame-shift, and use many other tactics to do nothing. They are in a constant state of "comfort-first" living. Their ultimate comfort always comes before the mission.

"And remember, it is a message to obey, not just to listen to. So don't fool yourselves. For if a person just listens and doesn't obey, he is like a man looking at his face in a mirror; as soon as he walks away, he can't see himself anymore or remember what he looks like. But if anyone keeps looking steadily into God's law for free men, he will not only remember it but he will do what it says, and God will greatly bless him in everything he does."

James 1:22-25 TLB

"You didn't choose me! I chose you! I appointed you to go and produce lovely fruit always, so that no matter what you ask for from the Father, using My name, He will give it to you." John 15:16

God depends on us to do what He has created us to do. Once again, many people are involved in our assignments and overall mission. What He has for us to do is more important than our comfort zones and earthly pleasures.

What a human being is "willing" to do or "not willing to do" is a visible statement of who they are and their value on the mission and the teams and individuals involved.

His Plan vs Our Plan

God created us. He designed us intentionally and on purpose with a specific mission that involves many assignments along the way. It's crucial to remember that it's His plan, not ours.

The scriptures reinforce and validate that He created, chose, and developed us from birth to accomplish our specific assignments.

When I share my story and my faith and speak on addiction and recovery across the USA, I make sure that they know precisely why God has chosen them. I know early in my recovery no one told me what I've learned over the past 24 years in recovery and as a young Christian.

When humans understand that their hearts are formed and developed through heartache, pain, and love, we can only begin to understand our calling and mission. As we feel pain, experience injustice, and give and receive love, these experiences develop our hearts and minds for our specific mission. I believe it's all intentional and on purpose.

Full Access to the Kingdom

God's kingdom lives through the power of the Holy Spirit inside us as believers and followers of Christ. Having full access to the hearts and minds of those God seeks is the greatest gift a Christ follower can ever ask for.

God's Kingdom is meant for me to live out NOW. When I live it, others experience the Kingdom through me, and I experience the Kingdom's blessings, freedom, power, true life, and purpose. When we lead our lives from a Kingdom Perspective utilizing the keys that grant us access into the hearts, minds, and souls of those God leads us to, it's then and only then that we experience the fullness of God's promises in our lives.

Without releasing control, we will never achieve FULL ACCESS to the Kingdom of God. We must understand and accept that His calling on our lives and the assignments He needs us to accomplish is extremely important. His calling on our lives involves so much more than us. His calling is linked explicitly to many others who need to experience His love flowing through us. He already has specific people that He needs us to engage with.

It's important to remember that Full Access to the Kingdom is Full Access to those God is seeking. They are the true treasure.

"Instead, be concerned above everything else with the Kingdom of God and with what He requires of you, and He will provide you with all these other things."

Matthew 6:33 GNV

"The heart of man plans his way, but the Lord establishes his steps."

Proverbs 16:9 ESV

When we master the art of allowing Him to lead every step of every day, we will accomplish the mission. God will arrange many things to ensure one specific conversation takes place.

God controls the game, whether you believe it or not. How we play is up to us. When we surrender to His army, we become one with His team from that moment on. He wins the game. The most incredible adventure begins once we understand that the game is not about us but what He can do through us.

Fishers of Men - Hot Spots

During my early years as a new Christian, I reached a point where I knew I needed to start sharing my faith. I had no idea where to begin, and my memories of all who had attempted to share their faith with me over the years were not good.

My first experience was when I was eight years old in Dermott, Arkansas, a tiny town. Two of my good friends were members of the local Pentecostal church. Their dad was a preacher there and extremely strict. They invited me to a revival one summer night.

I remember them showing a video of a man riding a motorcycle, and he went over a hill and had a wreck, and it showed his head getting cut off. Then, it immediately showed Satan with horns and a pitchfork standing in hell, burning. Many other kids and I ran to the front of the tent, terrified, and prayed with the pastor. When I got home that night, my mom went ballistic. That was my first experience with someone attempting to share their faith with me. I never knew what it meant. I had no idea who Jesus was or what the Bible or Gospel was.

As a young Christian working in a logistics center, I knew it was time to start sharing my faith. I needed to figure out where to begin. I knew the man on Beale Street in Memphis holding the sign yelling at me wasn't an option for me to use either.

While working in the Logistics Center, truck drivers would arrive to pick up loads of TVs and electronics. We would meet them at the front, escort them down the dock to their load, and count the items, and they would watch as we loaded. I thought, "This is a perfect opportunity to share my faith." I wasn't exactly sure where to begin. I knew I could get in trouble speaking about my faith to others at work.

One day, I decided to go for it. While escorting a rough-looking truck driver down the dock, I asked,

"Do you go to church?"

He replied, 'Yes, I actually have my own Church. I'm a Pastor.'

From that moment on, I was on fire. I asked every single one of them for years. These conversations were such high-energy encounters.

This was one of many experiences that proved to me beyond a shadow of a doubt the power of speaking up. These experiences also demonstrated that God leads us intentionally

"Jesus called out, 'Come along with me and I will show you how to fish for the souls of men!'" Matthew 4:19 TLB and precisely to people. If we don't speak up, we miss the immense blessings of experiencing the living God in real life.

As my faith intensified and the Fire within me grew hotter by the day, I concluded that I was called to reach more people.

I began seeking to identify what I call "Hot Spots." A hot spot is where many people need to feel God's love and where they are located.

Local jails, recovery centers, missions, community centers, bars, psychiatric hospitals, emergency rooms, and even places like Waffle House are all "Hot Spots."

God revealed to me the excitement and supernatural journey I will embark on when I "Go Get Them" instead of waiting for them to "Come to Me."

Since these fantastic revelations, my life has been the most exciting and fulfilling journey. I've met thousands of people I would've never met sitting at home in my comfort zone. Each encounter validates and confirms God's promises of how He intentionally leads us every step of the way.

When I receive calls from mothers weeping and desperately seeking help for their children, the mission is validated more and more.

"So here's what I want you to do, God helping you: Take your everyday, ordinary life—your sleeping, eating, going to work, and walking around life—and place it before God as an offering. Embracing what God does for you is the best thing you can do for him. Don't become so well-adjusted to your culture that you fit into it without thinking. Instead, fix your attention on God. You'll be changed from the inside out. Readily recognize what he wants from you and quickly respond to it. Unlike the culture around you, always dragging you down to its level of immaturity, God brings the best out of you and develops well-formed maturity in you."

Romans 12:1-2 The Message

> "Personal growth doesn't come from casting stones, but rather from helping others carry their burden." *Christopher Camp, Speaker Motivate With Coach Camp*

When I think about each individual God leads me to, I know, "They are ALL someone's child." They are also, most importantly, ALL God's children. That's precisely why He leads me to them: to help them discover His love for them and to help guide them into a better life free of man-made chemicals.

I love talking to strangers. Every single time I do, the moment I walk away, God lets me know I'm exactly where He wants me to be, doing exactly what He wants me to do! The adventure of following Christ far exceeds any other adventure in this life.

Surrender & Obedience

Following God wholeheartedly in this life requires many strengths, gifts, and personal characteristics.

Surrender to God's call on our lives is of extreme importance. We will never accomplish God's assignments if we are self-absorbed and live in a comfort-first mindset.

> "It takes a very special kind of person to willfully enter the pain of another person."
> *Dr. Theodore Bender, Ph.D., MD*

I know many incredible human beings that God has gifted immensely, and they only focus on their comfort. They worship sports, leisure, their families, the church, their careers, drugs and alcohol, and a variety of other things.

Obedience to God is also a learned skill. To walk in obedience, one must be very sensitive to the promptings of the Holy Spirit.

Instant obedience will teach you more in one experience than a lifetime of Bible studies.

As we grow as Christians and learn to follow Him wholeheartedly, He leads us through sanctification. The longer we follow Him, the more our faith is tested. As a result of His faithfulness, our faith continues to intensify and grow until we know that when He prompts us, we must act instantly. It becomes a natural response.

Enlarge my Territory

Recently, I prayed and asked God to expand my territory. I had always dreamed of sharing my story in jails, prisons, and recovery centers worldwide. And once again, God has made my wildest dreams a reality.

Today, I serve in multiple roles and spaces. As the Territory Manager for Woodland Recovery Center, I travel the entire North half of Mississippi and engage hundreds of organizations and individuals. My specific assignment is to build solid and lasting relationships with key leadership teams and decision-makers. The goal is to gain and sustain their trust and serve their organizations as they send me people struggling with addiction and mental health issues.

As a NAADAC - Nationally Certified Addiction Interventionist, I intervene in the lives of those struggling with addiction and alcoholism. NAADAC is the National Association for Alcoholism and Drug Abuse Counselors.

I am Certified Master Interventionist. I help people break free from the bonds of addiction and regain control of their lives. With over 20 years of experience in the field, I am passionate about helping people understand the underlying issues that lead to addiction and how to overcome them.

I also have the privilege of leading a weekly Christ-centered Alumni Zoom call with our current patients and graduates across the USA as part of my role with Bradford Health Services - Woodland Recovery Center.

As a Celebrate Recovery Inside - State Representative for North Mississippi and the Memphis Metro area, I assist in helping churches launch new CR Inside Ministries in jails and prisons in my Areas of Opportunity.

I've been speaking in local jails and prisons for over ten years. I lead Church and CR Inside in the DeSoto County Adult Detention Center twice weekly. I get to meet and engage those at rock bottom, share the love of Christ with them, and make sure they understand that they are called. I help them know that they, too, are God's Masterpiece. I teach them about free will, the Gospel, and activating God's promises.

My wife Stephanie began supporting a ministry in Uganda a few years back. Recently, I was asked to lead the Sunday morning Church service in Uganda via Zoom. Their smiles, applause, and hands raised did something in my heart that is unexplainable. This experience made me want to do more.

> "Understanding the importance of perseverance and determination by continuing to push forward, even faced with challenges, you will achieve greatness." *Stephanie Dodd, Realtor, CRI Ministry Leader*

As the Founder and CEO of the Hope Center of North Mississippi, I have the privilege of leading an Award-Winning Youth Mentorship Program. We mentor at-risk youth in 3rd-

12th grades. We are a Silver-Level Affiliate Partner of the Memphis Grizzlies Foundation. Our non-profit organization was nominated and awarded the Mentoring Program of the Year for the entire city of Memphis. In 2023, I was nominated and selected as the Mentoring Advocate of the Year. Our unique and futuristic mentoring model takes us to a whole new level of mentoring. We are touching numerous lives in our communities. Our next project is to obtain a space as a mentoring hub.

At this point, through platforms and organizations such as Facebook, Celebrate Recovery, Bradford Health Services, The Hope Center, and others, my story and God's story, which are the same, are being shared throughout the United States and worldwide.

Only a sovereign God could develop, sustain, and orchestrate the life I live today.

"We are ambassadors of the Anointed One who carry the message of Christ to the world, as though God were tenderly pleading with them directly through our lips."

2 Corinthians 5:20 TPT

I asked God once,

"Lord, how can You use me? I am a broken man?"

He replied,

"I am sending you to help other broken people. They cannot hear those who aren't broken, but they can hear you."

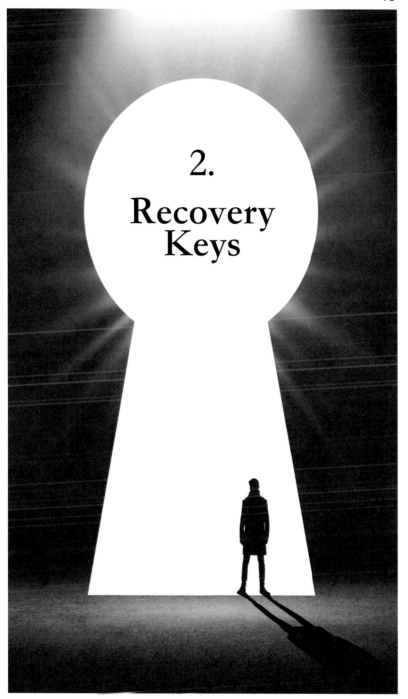

Today, I have over 24 years of successful recovery from the strongholds of addiction and alcoholism. I began experiencing the devastation of alcoholism at a very young age. My parents were divorced when I was two years old. In the early years of my life, my dad was an active alcoholic. As a result, I was raised by my single mother.

I began using cigarettes and alcohol at the age of 7, marijuana by the age of 11, and the usage progressed in high school. By the age of 33, I was a homeless addict in Joplin, Missouri, and eventually ended up in Memphis, Tennessee.

I hit rock bottom.

As always, God had other plans. My dad eventually quit drinking and was my very best friend in the whole world. At the end of my addiction, he would come and find me no matter where I was. He would always tell me,

"I believe in you, son. I know you can do it."

One of my deepest regrets is that my dad never got to see me clean. He taught me what I believe to be the most valuable life lessons that I get to "pay forward" and "teach others" every day in all the roles I serve.

My dad taught me this priceless lesson by his example. The lesson was how he loved ALL of his kids and his family. His UNCONDITIONAL love was what I've never forgotten, and it was the lesson that God has used to teach me the most about Himself. A parent's love for their children is the closest representation of God's love for ALL His children we will ever experience on earth.

When we refuse to give up on a human being, that experience is stored deep within their hearts and minds forever. They will remember the grace shown to them, and when the time comes to pay that grace forward, they will.

Recently, one of our program graduates called me. She said,

"Mr. Stacy, I can't believe you came and got me five times."

I said, "Actually, I came and got you 25 times. Every single morning when I arrived at the facility at 6:30 a.m. for work, you were running down the hill yelling and screaming."

The key takeaway is that she didn't remember the building, the groups, the food, or any of those issues. She remembered that I never gave up on her. She said, "You never gave up on me." That was what she remembered above all else. She called to thank me and tell me that she is now clean and doing well. She lives in South Texas and has regained custody of her five children.

> *"Addiction is the only disease in which we blame the person." Dr. Ted Bender, Ph.D., MBA*

These calls, text messages, and social media posts are priceless. Money and power can't buy these most precious treasures. I print and save all of these messages. These are messages that God lays on their hearts and minds. I don't ask them to write them. They do so on their own free will. They do so as they are humble and thankful. The truly humble are the ones who speak up and are transparent and vulnerable.

I'm extremely transparent and humble when I lead the weekly Christ-centered Recovery Zoom calls and the weekly Church services at the Recovery Center and the Jail. When I set the stage by sharing my most intense struggles and my love for them, they remember these things. I also ensure they know how important they are to God and that He has a purpose for them. I make it a point to ensure them that He wants to use them and their pain to help others.

While serving in multiple roles across the USA today, I travel in person to Hospitals, Intensive Care Units, Behavioral Health Centers, Addiction Recovery Centers, Psychiatric and Acute Care Hospitals, Homeless Shelters, Jails, Prisons, Drug Courts, Circuit Courts, Churches, the Streets, and even to the woods many times to personally engage and intervene in the lives of those God sends across my path.

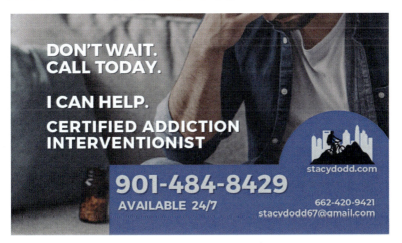

I have the BEST role in the Universe. What I GET to do every single day is a direct calling from God and a precious gift.

God revealed to me long ago that it's my responsibility to "Go Get Them." I'm not supposed to sit in my comfort zone and wait for them to find me. If you think about it, it's hard for God to lead someone that's using. So, it only makes sense for me to find them as He leads me.

I believe God is intentional and precise. I believe He leads me directly to those who need to feel and experience His love and those he's seeking.

I believe He speaks directly to them through me. Through my good and bad life experiences, I believe He's specifically equipped me for this mission.

When my phone rings, as it does 24 hours a day, seven days a week, I view each call as a call from God himself. I always answer, and I will go to places and do things most in my field wouldn't ever consider.

Personal Experience

In my first book, "Backpack to the 'Burbs," I describe my life as an addict and hitting a hard rock bottom. If you have not read this book, I encourage you to grab a copy from Amazon or ask for it at your local Books A Million.

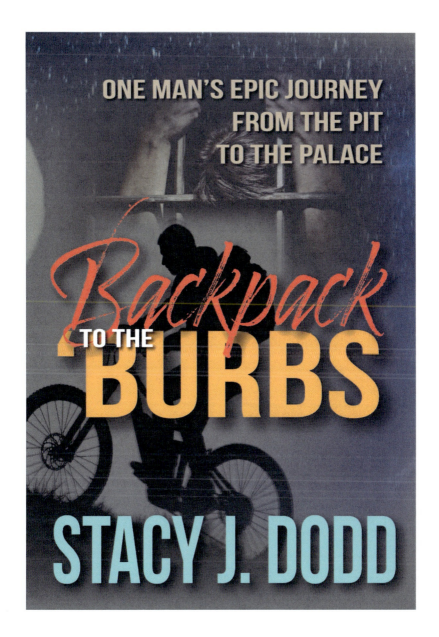

The Art of Communication with the Broken

I was blessed to have an Executive Coach early in my executive leadership career. She challenged me to rise higher and helped me reach my full potential. She also helped me recognize gifts that I already had and understand the magnitude of my calling.

Most people can't accept that God exists and that His spiritual principles are at work in our lives as He directs our daily paths. They were working to see how I was so successful concerning operations, my relationships with my team, and the patients I served and cared for.

I was asked the question:

"Without saying the word "God," describe what you do each day at the Recovery Center as you engage and lead your team."

My first thoughts were,

"Why in the world would I ever want to exclude God from anything?"

It took me a while to come up with an answer. This question prompted me to think about and investigate what I did and why.

Working in an Addiction Recovery Center is the experience of a lifetime. It's one of those experiences that can't be explained adequately. It's an experience that must be lived to understand adequately.

My final answer:

"I've Mastered the Art of Communication with the Broken."

As I was at the facility usually 12 hours per day, I would walk the halls constantly, speak at the Graduation Ceremonies, share my testimony regularly, and lead the weekly Church services on Sundays. I was in constant communication with approximately 200 patients and team members daily.

When monitoring the halls in the facility, my message to all I encountered was, "How's everything going? Is everyone being good to you? If you need anything, let me know. I love you!" This was my message to those I was responsible for serving and caring for and the Team Members I was responsible for serving and leading.

My leadership style was 'Love First." I had some young, inexperienced leaders who considered this leadership style as weak. I've discovered that it all depends on who you are leading. Organizations spend a fortune financially, have incredibly high turnover rates, poor customer service, and overall chaos when not using the "Love First" leadership style,

The "Control-Based," "Tough Guy," and "We Aren't Friends" worldly leadership style is the single most costly operations mindset in today's culture. If you pay close attention to HR staffing and internal costs, turnover costs, low morale, and loss of reputation within the community, you will find the root cause.

I always return to the operating style of Chick-fil-A®. They understand that understaffing is unacceptable when caring for people. You never hear, "We don't have your sandwich because someone called in sick today."

It's because they operate according to Integrity-Based Leadership. I describe this leadership style in the Leadership Keys section of this book. I love this topic.

Community Trust & Support

As with any endeavor involving serving others in this life, one must develop, maintain, and sustain trust. Trust is built through Integrity. One can cover up many things internally but can't cover up or manipulate one's reputation.

I've built a solid reputation over the years since my life transformation.

I have a reputation built on daily interactions and relationships with community and executive-level leaders from all walks of life.

As a Director on the Southaven Chamber of Commerce Board of Directors, I engage top executive-level leaders of organizations and corporations such as Fed-Ex World Headquarters, Baptist Hospital, State Farm Insurance, Edward Jones Investments, Tanger Outlets, Northwest Community College, and many more.

I have personal relationships with these amazing men and women. Sitting on the Board with them and engaging in conversations, I often wonder, " How did I end up here?" How did I end up with top-level executive leaders?"

God's intentional and precise leading is the truth about

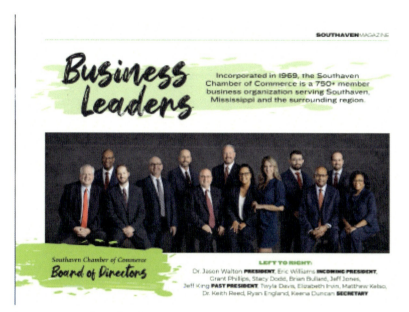

how I ended up in this place. And the most fantastic aspect is that they love me and treat me like their family. Unlike many top executive leaders who are grandiose and arrogant, these leaders know about my past and love me even more because I didn't give up. I often wonder how I ended up in Mississippi in this lifetime. It was the plan God had for me.

As with every other aspect of my life, it's not about me. It's all about what He can do in and through me as His love flows naturally through those walking in the Spirit into this Universe.

"If you must choose, take a good name rather than great riches; for to be held in loving esteem is better than silver and gold."

Proverbs 22:1 TLB

> "There are many quotes, books, videos, coaches, and classes on becoming a leader. It begins with a mindset of servitude and continues with a deep passion for people. Leaders are always leaders. Leaders do the hard things no one else cares to do on a consistent basis. They pour into others and share all the things, knowledge, support, and experience. They desire to leave everything better than they found it, their attitude, their companies, their environment, and their co-workers which becomes their legacy." *Debbie King, Executive Director - Southaven Chamber of Commerce, President - Southaven Rotary*

One of my GREATEST MEMORIES will always be how I used to think of top community leaders. Before my transformation, I used to think they all thought they were better than me, that they looked down on me, and that I was not good enough. When I first began leading in the community, I would be at the Chamber of Commerce Luncheons and watch the Mayor; I would think, "I wish he would speak to me." I wanted to be included.

Today, DeSoto County has four incredible men serving as Mayor. We have the Southaven Mayor, Darren Musselwhite; the Horn Lake Mayor, Allan Latimer; and the Olive Branch

Mayor, Ken Adams.

And guess what? I'm personal friends with each of them, and I have many pictures FROM LOCAL EVENTS WITH THEM.

They treat me with respect. They understand and accept me for who I am. They include me often in community events, and they trust me and call me when their loved ones or community members need help overcoming addiction.

A few months ago, Southaven Mayor Darren Musselwhite and I met to discuss how we could work together to help those families and individuals struggling with addiction. The fentanyl epidemic was a top priority. Our First Responders are at times being called to the exact locations multiple times each week to revive overdose victims using Narcan.

Since our initial conversation, I've presented Woodland Recovery Center to over 80 First Responder teams in and around DeSoto County. I wanted to thank Mayor Musselwhite, Mayor Adams, Mayor Johnson, and Mayor Latimer for their support and willingness to move quickly from awareness to the solution.

As a result of our team efforts, multiple individuals are in recovery now, and families and futures are being restored.

We know how to help those struggling with addiction, and we have access to unlimited resources to help them. We also know how to engage in conversations to initiate the beautiful recovery journey.

Recovery Keys

The following was published on Facebook[1], along with an article in the DeSoto Times-Tribune[2] in which Southaven Mayor Darren Musselwhite validates me and our mission. Articles like this validate and encourage me to keep going when times get tough. I'm so thankful to Mayor Musselwhite for his friendship, trust, and support of our mission.

Public Trust is a Master Key!

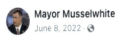

Mayor Musselwhite
June 8, 2022

FIGHTING DRUG ADDICTION...

"We have to do something more. We can't just keep reviving the same people with Narcan until the day we are too late!" is what I said after receiving daily Police and Fire EMS reports for responses to the same residences multiple times to revive the same overdose victims.

Parents of overdose victims contacted me and asked me to help after their children finally took the wrong pill with too much fentanyl. I'm just the Mayor of a Mississippi city. What can I do about a global problem? I sadly listened and thought about my own kids. I listened more and started asking more and more questions. I've never used drugs nor been addicted. I needed to listen even more and understand.

So I did and I learned...drug addiction knows no social or economic boundaries. It's no reflection on the addict's parents, school, church, team, or any other affiliation, with the exception of the one who introduces the drugs the first time. Dangerous drugs are everywhere in our world now. Drug addiction can happen to anyone. Read this again and know...it can happen to your kids and grandkids. Overdose deaths since 2020 are the highest in U.S. history.

Then, I heard the life story of a man named Stacy Dodd. Stacy is a 20-plus year recovered drug addict who lived for many years homeless on the streets of Joplin, Missouri. Who could be better to help save the life of a struggling drug addict than a former struggling drug addict who overcame the addiction and lived? So, I met with him and asked him to explain drug addiction in detail to me and how to save people. I won't try to tell his story like he can tell it, other than to say this...he knows how to beat drug addiction, why he was given a second chance, and is willing to spend the rest of his life helping others do the same.

This message is not about me as I've done nothing but act as a small conduit. Instead, it's about sharing the reality of the dangers of drug addiction and sharing a real solution of a God-sent man who's committed his life to this cause. If you know someone in danger, please see the contact information in the shared post.

---

[1] https://www.facebook.com/MayorMusselwhite/posts/pfbid0BR8WvoSLDVzksWqsxr1hTwB5GWWKUqBnkC66ZMtvV6u1nfUWXNVTNBh4YrWXDdvPl
[2] https://www.desototimes.com/news/drug-counselor-helping-southaven-deal-with-drug-addiction/article_f6f8ff98-6065-11ec-80ba-5f152b720e94.html

Drug counselor helping Southaven deal with drug addiction

By Mark Randall Dec 19, 2021

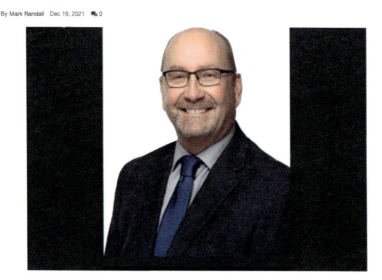

Southaven Mayor Darren Musselwhite has heard a lot of stories over the years from parents and residents who have lost a loved one or somebody they know due to a drug overdose, or are dealing with a family member or friend struggling with addiction.

In 2021, the United States reached a grim milestone. For the first time in its history, deaths from drug overdoses topped 100,000 deaths, exceeding the number of people killed in motor vehicle accidents.

Musselwhite said the city's fire, police, and EMS personnel respond to overdose calls almost daily - some to the same address in the same week.

"They administer NARCAN and then they are called back again and the same person is deceased," Musselwhite said. "So a lot of times it's not if they are going to die, it's when."

Rather than sit back feeling helpless to stop the problem, Musselwhite recently reached out to Stacy Dodd, who is the regional ambassador for Vertava Health, a drug and alcohol addiction treatment center, about helping the city to be more proactive in dealing with heroin and other drug addictions in an effort to save more lives.

Dodd is a former drug addict who has been clean for more than 20 years. He wrote about his life as an addict in his book "Backpack to the Burbs" and has been sharing his story and offering encouragement to addicts to help them get their lives back.

"His mission is to keep people from experiencing the bad things that he experienced," Musselwhite said. "He wants to save lives. He knows what these people are going through and he wants to help them."

Musselwhite said Dodd has agreed to partner with the city and has been meeting with first responders to talk about the services that Vertava Health provides and to make himself available 24/7 to help out in drug overdose situations.

"We have brought him in to all our fire stations to meet our personnel," Musselwhite said. "He's even offered to give his cell phone number out to anyone on the spot when our personnel come in to contact with someone who is dangerously addicted. He's reaching out his hand and will help them. He will respond to them. He will counsel them. He will try to help them."

Musselwhite commended Dodd for offering to help and said he hopes the effort will be a liaison between not doing anything for people suffering from addictions, to getting them the resources they need to save their life.

"I think it is an awesome thing," Musselwhite said. "We are not just sitting back and watching people die. We are doing all we can to save their lives. We look forward to what he can accomplish."

Dodd said he is glad that Musselwhite reached out to him. Drug overdoses - particularly from Fentanyl - are a big problem in DeSoto County that is only getting worse.

"Mayor Musselwhite has really stood up and taken the lead on this," Dodd said. "He really cares about the community. I told him I would earn his trust, would build his trust, and that I would maintain his trust."

Dodd said he helps educate first responders about drug addiction, but mostly informs them about the services that Vertava Health provides and where addicts can go to get help.
"I teach them about our program and I tell them about our doctors and give them the information about our program. Nothing is going to be okay until they quit using the chemicals. So we have to get them somewhere to get the chemicals out of there. Once we can get rid of the chemicals, then lives miraculously turn around."

Dodd had some information cards printed that he gives to first responders with his phone number on it so addicts can get in touch with him.

"Whenever the first responders go out to the scene, they have these cards," Dodd said. "They're not saying to call Vertava. They are just saying that if you want help, these people can help you."

He said although Vertava Health requires insurance or private pay, he can help direct addicts to programs and resources to get treatment.

"My passion is to help people," Dodd said. "I have families and people of all different income levels. I have people who have a lot of money and people who have little money call me all the time. What's different about us is if you call me and you know your son is overdosing and you don't know what to do, I know what to do. And there are a lot of programs for funding for people who don't have insurance. I just try and steer them to resources that are already in place."

Dodd said he used his own experience as a former drug addict to connect with people who are currently struggling to get them the help they need to turn things around.

"The person that is addicted is going to have to go to treatment," Dodd said. "But if we can save one or two lives in each city in DeSoto County every week, then that's 100 to 200 people a year."

Recovery Solutions

My lifetime of active addiction and over 24 years of walking a successful recovery has led me to much insight and the discovery of solutions. I know what works and what doesn't work.

Over the past twenty years, my roles as a Celebrate Recovery State Representative and Celebrate Recovery Inside State Representative for North Mississippi and the Memphis Metro Area have given me much hands-on experience.

Over the past ten years, my multiple roles with Bradford Health Services –Woodland Recovery Center have given me incredible experience and insight.

My roles include Certified Peer Support Specialists, Certified Peer Support Specialists -Supervisor, Director of Operations, Area Vice President of Operations, Community Ambassador, Business Development, Account Executive, and Territory Manager.

As an executive-level leader with Bradford, I was privileged to have up close and personal experience with all aspects of the addiction recovery space.

I worked closely with the clinical and medical teams on all operations. I was trained and experienced with all safety compliance operations. As a fully accredited Substance Use and Mental Health facility, we are licensed by the Mississippi Department of Mental Health, the Joint Commission, and CARF.

I was fully equipped and trained in all my roles and given

a Master's Level of education via hands-on experience working closely with the Top Executive leaders within our organization across the USA. I was honored to be equipped with the very best in the addiction recovery space.

My multiple roles leading within the Church as an Ordained Minister, Life Groups Director, Celebrate Recovery Ministry Leader, Celebrate Recovery State Representative, Celebrate Recovery Inside State Representative, and DeSoto County Adult Detention Center Jail Ministry Leader provided me with much insight and experience.

When it comes to Addiction, Alcoholism, and Christ-centered recovery, I know what works and what doesn't.

I've had personal relationships with over 12,000 men and women admitted to our Woodland Recovery Center addiction treatment program, the honor of baptizing over 800 patients, and the privilege of leading thousands to Christ in the CR Inside jail and prison ministry. In my current role with Bradford Health Services, I receive hundreds of calls weekly.

In 2014, I walked into an old hotel, just seeking to encourage those in recovery that they could make it. Little did I know that I would fall in love with the most amazing people on the planet. During our Grand Opening Ceremony, I asked my Pastor to come to the facility and pray over me and the facility. I'll never forget his words:

"God just gave you the most powerful ministry in DeSoto County."

He was right. More healing and transformations occur at this facility today than anywhere else in the region.

I believe the ultimate solution to addiction and alcoholism is a precise combination of treatment strategies followed by a lifetime of daily spiritual aftercare and maintenance.

The ultimate combination that delivers the best long-term outcomes is the professionals' excellent medical and clinical care. Add a solid spiritual foundation, followed by a lifetime of spiritual care, accountability, and service.

Surrender to Win

When I speak on addiction and recovery, there are a few things to always keep in mind. Addiction and alcoholism are the same thing. I hear so many say, "I drink, but I'm not an addict or drug user."

For the record, alcohol is the worst. Alcohol is referred to as "cunning and baffling" in the Big Book of Alcoholics Anonymous. When I encounter those struggling with alcohol, they are sure they are just fine. They're only hurting themselves and can quit anytime they wish. The only problem is that "none of this is true."

When I speak on addiction and recovery, I make sure to confirm that it doesn't matter how rich you are, how smart you are, or how good-looking you are; you will never win.

Addiction is the only battle in life in which we, "SURRENDER TO WIN"

Free Will & Man-Made Chemicals

When I speak on addiction and recovery across the USA over the years, my message has developed over time as I continue to learn, grow, and witness the struggles, solutions, and outcomes. The long-term outcomes always deliver the truth.

When I describe free will, I always do so in a way that those I'm speaking to can fully understand. I'm a big fan of Christ-centered recovery, which has driven my successful recovery and experiencing my best life.

I always use this message in recovery centers, jails, and prisons.

"Does everyone in this room have Anger, Lust, Pride, Jealousy and Selfishness?"

They all always agree, and at that time, I say,

"Say it with me. I admit I'm a sinner."

Then I continue.

"Have you ever done something you knew you shouldn't do, and you've done it repeatedly?

And you wake up, just you and God, maybe a tear coming down your face, and say, 'I'm Sorry, God.'

You're not just sorry so you can continue using, but are you truly sorry?"

They always agree.

Then I say,

"Say it with me. I repent of my sins."

The message continues:

"In the Beginning, God created man and woman, placed them in the garden, and told them, 'You can have everything beautiful in this life forever, but don't touch that tree.' You and God know your tree. One will never have the beautiful life God has for us and eat from our tree simultaneously."

The two can't co-exist. We must pick one. If we refuse to pick one, there will be chaos within our souls.

When we surrender our lives to Christ, the Holy Spirit takes up permanent residence in the believer's body. From that moment on, we embark on the journey of Sanctification, and God works in and through us as mobile vessels of His love.

Through the power of the Holy Spirit, His love and gifts flow directly through us into the lives of all He leads across our path.

I believe God calls them from their old lives into a new life with Him.

Recovery Keys 67

If they refuse to surrender, pay attention to the red flags, and head back down that old road, God will jack them up. They will experience financial and family problems. Things like getting beat up, robbed, car wrecks, jail stays, legal issues, self-esteem issues, and so on will continue.

God will not stop seeking them. They will not win until they surrender.

It seems like punishment, but it's a great honor. He wants to use them, seek them relentlessly, and have them work for Him.

And unlike most prisoners, they become one of the team when they surrender to Him.

From that moment on, all the promises in His word belong

to them. They don't need to have it all figured out. He already does.

If we put our faith in God, no more chemicals, tell the truth, and go to work, our wildest dreams will come true.

Recently, our Pastor challenged us with this question.

"What would you do if you could not fail?"

I present this same challenge to them. I also remind them that "it must be legal." As long as we stay clean, no drugs and alcohol, put our faith in God, tell the truth, and go to work, we will not fail. God needs us to accomplish the calling He has placed on our lives. He will ensure that we succeed. We must trust Him.

When you see someone in recovery trying extra hard, many times, they are trying to build the life they missed out on as a result of their addiction. Some things are their fault, and some probably not. Don't judge. Most times, they have experienced enough of that. They know their imperfections. They've tasted shame and regret. Give them a hand up without enabling. It is possible. Help them succeed, tell them you love them unconditionally, and never throw in the towel. They are all someone's child. This mindset can change the world. You are not remembered for what you achieved. You are remembered for what you survived!

Enabling

My extensive and hands-on experience with enabling

began at a very young age. As a single mother raised me, she did her best. As a Registered nurse anesthetist, she worked long hours seven days a week and was always on call. As a latch-key kid, I was home alone most of the time. My first enabling memories were when my mom would leave two 20-dollar bills on the table each morning so I would have money for food and school. Little did she know, that was enough for everything I needed, plus cigarettes and marijuana. Fast forward to age 33, and I lived in the woods just North of Joplin, Missouri, addicted to methamphetamine.

My mom would send me an envelope with $300 cash twice a month. This supplied my ever-growing and extensive addiction.

One evening, my mom and stepdad diligently located an Al-Anon meeting they were going to attend in their attempt to help me. On their way to the meeting in downtown Memphis, they got lost. I believe that, because of God's intentional leadership, they ended up at another meeting. The group members stopped the meeting that night and told my parents their testimonies.

The following day, at 8 am, I received a call from my mom. She said,

"Don't you ever call me again and ask me for any money until you get your life straightened up."

That's what moms do. They never give up. She never gave up on me.

My mom's first act of "Tough Love" was the game changer in my life.

> It was only when she stopped enabling me that God was able to intervene directly.
>
> Remember, man-made chemicals annihilate our free will.

At this point, I had an addiction that required a large amount of drugs daily. My addiction required a lot of money. When she stopped sending the money, the addiction remained. At that point, I went deeper into my addiction, and I landed in a very dark place.

Today, as an Addiction Interventionist, a Celebrate Recovery State Representative, and a Territory Manager for Bradford Health Services, I encounter all levels of enabling in real life on the front lines of the battle against addiction.

I will say that moms are the worst. Their unconditional love for their children leads to them feeling responsible for them. When you add co-dependency and other internal issues, the result is often devastating.

An important thing to remember is that when the addict or alcoholic is allowed to make the decisions, the decisions will always be made that will enable them to continue using and maintain their lifestyle.

It's also important to remember that …

> It's impossible to help someone who won't participate in their own rescue.

My personal and professional experience taught me that money is the critical root of all enabling. I've included some key facts on enabling and addiction.

Am I an Enabler?

Family and friends try to protect their loved one from financial or legal consequences, but that often has the unintended effect of enabling the substance abuse to worsen. People in early recovery typically need emotional and material support. This support is helpful and healthy, but it's essential to let them know you will only be supporting their recovery efforts – nothing else. Focus on helping your loved one's healthy future goals, such as continuing education or finding a job.

Signs of Addiction

- Loss of control: Drinking or drugging more than a person wants to, for longer than they intended, or despite telling themselves it will not happen again.

- Neglecting other activities: spending less time on activities that used to be important (hanging out with family and friends, exercising hobbies or other interests) because of the use of alcohol or drugs; drop in attendance and performance at work or school

- Risk-taking: more likely to take serious risks to obtain

one's drugs of choice

- Relationship issues: People struggling with addiction are known to act out against those closest to them, particularly if someone is attempting to address their substance abuse problems, complaints from co-workers, supervisors, teachers, or classmates

- Secrecy: Going out of one's way to hide the amount of drugs or alcohol consumed or one's activities when drinking or drugging unexplained injuries or accidents.

- Changing appearance: Serious changes in appearance or deterioration of hygiene or physical appearance – lack of showering, slovenly appearance, unclean clothes

- Family History: A family history of addiction can dramatically increase one's predisposition to substance abuse

- Tolerance: Over time, a person's body adapts to a tolerance to the point that they need more and more of it to have the same reaction

- Withdrawal: As the effect of the alcohol or drugs wears off, the person may experience symptoms such as anxiety or jumpiness, shakiness or trembling, sweating, nausea and vomiting, insomnia, depression, irritability, fatigue or loss of appetite, headaches

- Continued use: Despite negative consequences, even though it is causing problems on the job, with relationships, or health, a person continues drinking and drugging.

Physical Signs May Include:

- Over-active or under-active (depending on the drug)
- Repetitive speech patterns
- Dilated pupils, red eyes
- Excessive sniffing and runny nose (not attributable to a cold)
- Looking pale or undernourished
- Clothes do not fit the same
- Weight loss
- Change in eating habits
- Unusual odors or body odor due to a lack of personal hygiene
- Behavioral Signs May Include:
- Missing work/school
- Work/school problems
- Missing important engagements

- Isolating/secretive about activities

- Disrupted sleep patterns

- Legal problems

- Relationship/marital problems

- Financial problems (e.g., always needing money)

- Conversations dominated by using or drug/alcohol-related topics

- Emotional Irritability/Argument

- Defensiveness

- Inability to deal with stress

- Loss of interest in activities/people that used to be part of their lives

- Obnoxious

- Silly

- Confused easily

- Denial Rationalizing – Offering alibis, excuses, justifications, or other explanations for their using behavior.[1]

The decision to stop enabling is one of the hardest

---

[1] (n.d.). FAQ. Https://www.Stacydodd.com. Retrieved August 29, 2024, from https://www.stacydodd.com/faq

decisions a human will ever make. The decision-making process should be based on the following facts:

What's going to happen if I stop enabling?

What could happen if I don't?

In my life, it was only when my mom stopped enabling that true transformation and healing began.

Skills - DBT

My first exposure to Dialectical Behavioral Skills took place when I met Bobby Scott, LMFT, CANADA, C-DBT. He is a DBT expert and owns his own private practice, Bobby Scott & Associates Professional Counseling in Southaven, Mississippi.

Bobby hired me in 2015 at Turning Point Recovery. I'd never even heard of DBT. Over the next decade, I've witnessed the transformational power of DBT when applied in the lives of those struggling with Substance Use Disorders. The skills are priceless.

By teaching those struggling with alcoholism and addiction how to identify, manage, and control their emotions, all aspects of their lives are positively impacted. DBT delivers long-term positive outcomes in our relationships. Our careers,

families, ministries, friendships, and our leadership are all enhanced when we learn how to respond to our emotions with positive outcomes.

Our unique model at Woodland Recovery Center consists of medical, clinical, spiritual, and long-term aftercare programming. Our core modality in DBT. IT is at the center of living our best life and reaching our full potential.

The DBT skills assist in helping us respond strategically to deliver positive outcomes, help me daily with my relationships, family, ministry, and mentorship, as well as with my mental health, as I strive to have a balanced life.

I strongly encourage you to investigate and give DBT a try. These skills have been and continue to be life-changing for me.

Without going into detail on the exact therapy procedures, I will offer an introduction to an article I found on Psychology Today's website that explains it best.

Dialectical behavior therapy (DBT) is a structured program of psychotherapy with a strong educational component designed to provide skills for managing intense emotions and negotiating social relationships. Originally developed to curb the self-destructive impulses of chronic suicidal patients, it is also the treatment of choice for borderline personality disorder, emotion dysregulation, and a growing array of psychiatric conditions. It consists of group instruction and individual therapy sessions, both conducted weekly for six months to a year,

The "dialectic" in dialectical behavior therapy is an acknowledgment that real life is complex, and health is not a static thing but an ongoing process hammered out through a continuous Socratic dialogue with the self and others. It is continually aimed at balancing opposing forces and investigating the truth of powerful negative emotions.

DBT acknowledges the need for change in a context of acceptance of situations and recognizes the constant flux of feelings—many of them contradictory—without having to get caught up in them. Therapist-teachers help patients understand and accept that thought is an inherently messy process. DBT is itself an interplay of science and practice.[1]

To find out more about DBT skills and process, visit: https://www.psychologytoday.com/us/therapy-types/dialectical-behavior-therapy

---

[1] (n.d.). Dialectical Behavior Therapy. Https://www.Psychologytoday.com. Retrieved August 29, 2024, from https://www.psychologytoday.com/us/therapy-types/dialectical-behavior-therapy

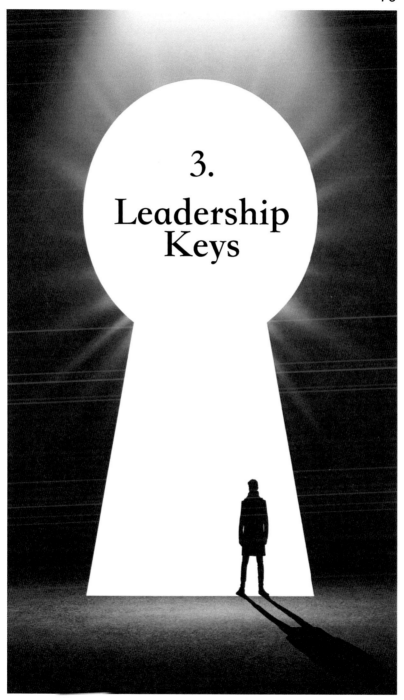

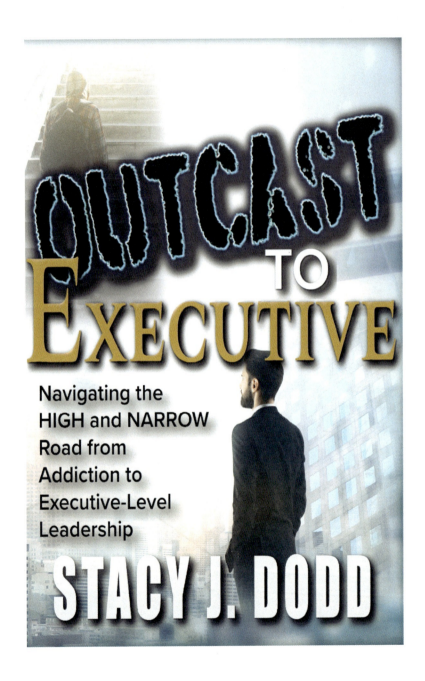

In my second book, "Outcast to Executive," I share the incredible leadership lessons I've learned in multiple leadership roles. The memories of my first roles as a supervisor for a global logistics corporation, my role as a Life Groups Director and Celebrate Recovery Ministry Leader, and then on to Director of Operations and eventually the CEO/Area Vice President for a National Healthcare Organization, and my role as the CEO and Founder of the award-winning youth mentorship program are so special. God led me to what I still believe: the very BEST leaders in the business. I was led by Clinical Psychologists, Medical Doctors, CEO's, and Mayors.

To kick off this section on Leadership Keys, I'm sharing the foreword from my second book, Outcast to Executive, which my amazing Executive Coach wrote.

"Key principles of leadership are regularly touted, directed, dissected, espoused, professed, taught, and blogged upon. We read countless articles and the latest business books on what it takes to be a good leader. But the real learning is when we get to see it in action, or better yet experience the transformative power of working for a true leader. For those who have had the opportunity to work with Stacy Dodd they have been witness to best of these principles in practice.

Leadership is built through a keen understanding of vision and purpose. That unique ability to create energy and alignment around the day to day activities, then to tie those back so that they embody the purpose and edge an organization ever closer to its vision. Coupled with a grass roots perspective on deep contribution to the human condition, Stacy's impact in the recovery community can't be understated. But what might be missed is the daily self work over many years that he dedicates towards being the best leader possible.

Welcoming feedback and ideas, speaking truth when it's hard, and holding onto a deeply rooted trust in a power greater than himself aids in his finding direction, assurance and clarity. While these are hallmarks, they are not exclusive to his path.

Lessons in bravery, stories of humility, anecdotes of learning ones limits and gifts are interlaced with humor and curiosity. Through all of that it's important to understand that the journey, the path to today is never forgotten. It's more than a badge of honor woven from critical life lessons. It shapes itself into a humbling connection with a universe of people yet to serve, the infinite extension of his mission.

This book is a peak inside a work always in progress, always being refined as he himself, as a leader continues to stretch and grow. His willingness to challenge his skills and experience, to push himself beyond what's comfortable, in search of new ways to serve the vision embody the best lessons in leadership.

Beyond that he is proof that beyond addiction is a story yet to be written, an ongoing evolution of the human potential. Life is about what you make each day out of the lessons from your past and the vision for your future."

Carrie Cahill - Executive Coach

"...grab hold of your seats and hang on, kids, because the sky's the limit." - Chris Solaas, Author

"This book is a peek inside a work always in progress, continuously refined as (Stacy), as a leader, continues to grow." - Carrie Cahill, Executive Coach

In 2001, a Greyhound bus arrived in Memphis with a passenger. This passenger had nothing except a backpack with two changes of dirty clothes, a Bible that was gifted to him, and a pendant that he'd found in the alley in Joplin, Missouri. He was unsure of himself, ashamed of his past, and uncertain of his future.

Today, this same passenger is a corporate executive leader and social influencer.

So how did he go from a destructive lifestyle to becoming a successful executive? How did he overcome the stigma of being an outcast in society to a highly respected social influencer in his community?

This book is designed to emotionally, intellectually, and spiritually support and equip those overcoming challenges such as addiction, depression, low self-esteem, humiliation, insecurity, and all other struggles while attempting to rebuild their lives and careers in a vicious and highly competitive workforce.

It will help you identify the triggers of failure, manage your feelings and emotions, and allow them to drive your success instead of leading to failure, and most of all - not to give up on your dreams.

Stacy Dodd is an author, speaker, and executive leader who overcame drug addiction to become a respected community and corporate leader. His story starts with his book, **"Backpack to the 'Burbs"** and continues to unfold each day.
www.stacydodd.com

Integrity-Based Leadership

The truth is always the best answer. When I think of integrity-based leadership, Chick-fil-A® always comes to mind immediately. I had the privilege of touring their corporate headquarters in Atlanta, Georgia. Their energy and integrity stand out front and center. Giant signs with the words "Integrity," "Unassuming," "Honesty," etc. are everywhere.

> "Each person's destiny is not a matter of chance; It's a matter of choice. It's determined by what we say, what we do, and whom we trust." *S. Truett Cathy, Founder - Chick-fil-A®*

I've also had the personal experience of working with our local CFA Executive Leadership teams, Stuart Davidson and April Armstrong. I've witnessed these two individuals go above and beyond, as their lives are an example. They serve our community diligently and with integrity. They go above and beyond as they support their team members at work and in their personal struggles.

> "In times of doubt or anxiousness…Be Still…God's Got It! When you Don't Know….God Knows." *April Armstrong, Catering & Brand Development Director, Chick-fil-A® Southaven, Mississippi*

Chick-fil-A® doesn't seek to save money at the expense of its reputation. They don't short-staff or tolerate their customers being disrespected. The energy at all of their locations stands out in our culture today.

I believe ALL organizations in our world should follow their example.

When it comes to our personal leadership, total honesty must always come first. During the past two decades, I've encountered all types of leaders operating at all levels. When I encounter a human being in a top-level position who I know for a fact doesn't always tell the truth, I lose respect immediately.

The main issue with a human being that doesn't always tell the truth is, you never know when they're lying.

I remember it so vividly when I was first given a leadership role. My first thought was that I must always tell the truth. I was sure that if I ever got caught lying, that would disqualify me. I carry that mindset to this very day.

A few years back, one of my leaders stated,

"No matter how bad it got, you always told the truth."

Honesty is the first and non-negotiable expectation of a leader. One shouldn't be allowed to lead if they don't always tell the truth. Some of the most dishonest leaders I've ever met held the highest-ranking positions. To me, the pastor, doctor, CEO, etc., should be the ones with the highest levels of integrity. Remember, true integrity requires 100% honesty at all times. There is no middle ground with honesty.

As leaders, we can activate the gifts and bring out the best in those we lead. By validating and believing in them, we can be the vessel God uses to light their fire and push them to rise to the next level in His calling on their lives.

Cultural Competence

My first experiences learning about Cultural Competence were initiated during my relationship with the Memphis Grizzlies Foundation. As a Silver-Level Affiliate, we have access to on-going trainings. I have even had the privilege and honor of leading the "Elements of Effective Mentoring" training sessions.

Whether leading a youth mentoring program, church ministry, or an executive level team, cultural competence is game changing knowledge that will set you apart.

You have to experience and tap into the culture you wish to impact. You have to understand what touches the heart of the culture before the culture will respond to you. Culture will always respond and support you when they know you care enough to spend your precious time investing in them.

People have a built in sensor for authenticity. Once you win them over they're yours for life. That's when you witness a culture founded in LOVE. If I remember correctly, the

"The one who faithfully manages the little he has been given will be promoted and trusted with greater responsibilities. But those who cheat with the little they have been given will not be considered trustworthy to receive more." Luke 16:10 TPT greatest teacher of all time made that His #1 FOCUS.

When doing a Google search on the best definition of Cultural Competence, it states the following:

Cultural competence is the ability to understand and respect the differences in values, beliefs, and attitudes between cultures. It also involves the ability to respond appropriately to these differences in a variety of settings, including personal and professional.

Here are some examples of cultural competence in different fields:

<u>*Health care*</u>

Cultural competence in health care is the ability to provide services that meet the needs of patients from different cultures, including their social, cultural, and linguistic needs. This can help improve the quality of care and health outcomes, and reduce health disparities.

<u>*Social work*</u>

Cultural competence in social work involves being aware of how different cultural groups experience their uniqueness and deal with their differences and similarities. It also involves using an intersectionality approach to examine forms of oppression, discrimination, and domination.

Cultural competence is a developmental process that evolves over time. Individuals and organizations can be at different levels of awareness, knowledge, and skills on the cultural competence continuum.[1]

---
[1] (GOOGLE, 2024)

"Dear children, let's not merely say that we love each other; let us show the truth by our actions."

1 John 3:18 TLB

Action Activates

All of the knowledge in the Universe is fruitless without action. For example, one can read the Bible daily and recite it word for word, but if they don't do what the Word says, they will never experience the promises.

Our actions tell the truth about who we are. They are visible proof of our belief in and dedication to the mission and assignment.

We lose respect and influence when our actions don't match our words. As representatives of Christ on this earth, we should, at minimum, be honest.

A lack of integrity, laziness, arrogance, grandiosity, and entitlement stand out so much more in the life of a human being who publicly claims their identity in Christ.

I speak more on this topic in the "Great Christian Cover-Up" chapter.

I've learned that when you are willing to do what others are willing to do, I will have influence and outcomes others will not have.

Degree vs. Calling

I've experienced and engaged with multiple leadership styles and personalities throughout my career. Many of the worst leaders and bad human beings have held the highest degrees.

I've also discovered that when intense passion is present in the heart, mind, and energy of a human being on fire for the mission, that person will consistently outperform and outlast those with even the highest education levels and skill sets.

I've experienced the entitlement, arrogance, and grandiosity that often accompany those with college degrees' work ethic and performance.

While I would never discredit or minimize the hard work and dedication required to gain a degree, I will say that a degree doesn't deliver performance and long-term outcomes.

I've discovered that, as with every other aspect of life, when we follow the Kingdom Mindset, the long-term outcomes of success, efficiency, high energy, and passion are always present.

Through our life experiences, hardships, injustice, heartbreak, wins, and failures, God equips us for the mission and assignment of leadership.

A Degree from the Master will outlast, outperform, and deliver the long-term outcomes that a Master's Degree simply can't deliver.

As mentioned earlier, no force in the Universe has the power to deliver what the Holy Spirit of the living God can.

The passion, fire, energy, determination, discernment, conviction, joy, peace, contentment, kindness, and so much else that exists within the heart, mind, and soul of the spirit-filled believer can only be delivered through the power of the Holy Spirit.

No organization, book, church, degree, pastor, CEO, doctor, lesson, building, or group has that power. It's only through His spirit that these priceless gifts are delivered. The favor of God will always accomplish more with less.

Identifying the favor and presence of God that exists in the life and mission of a human being is the highest level of Kingdom-minded executive level leadership.

Communication

It's impossible to help someone who doesn't trust you. Building absolute trust with someone who doesn't know you is impossible. To know someone, you must spend time with them. Most leaders today are too busy focused on themselves and their ultimate comfort-first leadership styles to spend time with anyone they view as less than themselves. Many say they love them and care, but most times, it's fake. They say they care to keep their title and role but would never give someone struggling $1 of their own money if they were starving. You will learn the truth when you base your analysis on a person's actions. Talk is so cheap and deceiving.

In today's culture, a leader's action is the highest form of communication. A leader's example communicates more than words have the power to communicate.

Always know that those you lead watch you. They know if you genuinely care or are just putting on a show. Basic human instinct always reveals the truth. Always know that just because they don't say something doesn't mean they don't see the truth.

Many times in an attempt to outsmart others, men outsmart themselves.

Simplification

A lack of resources and support will lead a person into "survival mode."

The most outstanding leaders understand the importance of "Simplification."

One of my first lessons in Executive Leadership was, "Don't ever create tasks and assignments that you don't have the staffing and resources to accomplish."

Early in my leadership roles in healthcare, non-profit, and ministry, the resources and staffing simply weren't there.

This forced me to look inside for the answers. I discovered that unhappy people overcomplicate things and those who complain the most do the least.

When we simplify, we free up more time for the true mission of serving the patients, customers, and strangers God has entrusted us to serve.

> "Don't look for wealth in money, cars, homes, investments – Look for wealth in the things you give – love, time, encouragement, opportunities, acknowledgement, praise, compassion, empathy. These are the riches of life. Nothing is ever truly valuable until you give it away." *Martha Hudspeth Fondren, Grant & Company*

In today's culture, if you don't serve those God sends to you well, they will go elsewhere.

Validation

The most outstanding leaders I've ever known fully knew the unlimited power that lies in validation. The weakest leaders I've ever known would never validate. They are the ones who can't see past themselves long enough to spend time on those they've been entrusted to lead.

The leaders who refuse to validate only steal from themselves and the organizations they're responsible for leading.

Last year, I received this validation from a healthcare organization. It encouraged me to keep pushing, even through change and challenging times.

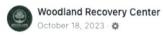

Leadership Styles

During my over twenty years in multiple leadership roles, I've experienced every leadership style. I've served under the best and the worst. The older I get and the more I experience, the more I discover that the best long-term outcomes are delivered when we follow the Kingdom Principles.

I will never be convinced that God's principles and promises aren't intended to be surrendered in the workplace and business. I've heard so many worldly-minded and immature leaders say, "It's business." I've even had one leader claim that one of the worst leaders I've ever known was a "Godly leader." I lost respect for this man immediately. This man will do anything to anyone for the right amount of money. This is not integrity-based leadership.

Early in my leadership career, I noticed the immense financial and operational consequences that organizations face when they lead according to worldly norms.

The Human Resources cost of high turnover, lawsuits, time away from work from unsatisfied team members, and the mental health impact of constant chaos are overwhelming.

I discovered that the "Love First" leadership style is the best choice. This style minimizes all of the above costs. Team members are happier, more creative, and more productive when they know they are loved.

> **True success is never about which team member outperforms or is superior to his or her teammates. True success is always about accomplishing the mission. The mission is always of supreme importance. Superior mindsets and relentless competition can cause harm to the team, morale, and performance. Those we seek and serve are why we do what we do. It's NEVER about us. It's ALWAYS about them.**

I've never understood how anyone can claim to love the patients or customers they serve but not equally love the team members who care for them. How can you work together daily under intense conditions and not care for each other?

This is another example of how worldly trends aren't the best and deliver secret consequences for the entire organization.

Dictator-type leaders exhibit control out of arrogance and boasting. They actually create a bad vibe for the entire organization.

It's not what you look at that matters; it's what you see. It's so apparent and straightforward to detect those that lead from a worldly point of view compared to those that lead from a Kingdom Perspective and operate according to proven scriptural principles.

In my over two decades in executive-level roles in multiple spaces, I've discovered that the very best long-term outcomes are achieved when we follow Godly principles.

The truth is that whether we are leading in the healthcare, non-profit, or ministry spaces, the same absolute truths remain. I will always stand by my solid belief that the "LOVE FIRST" leadership style will always deliver the best long-term outcomes.

Hire the Fire

When you "Hire the Fire," you can release these individuals, and they will deliver. If you trust them and truly believe God's spirit is directing every step as His word describes, you can sit back and enjoy the show.

Choosing who to hire and promote can make or break you as an Executive Leader. I've discovered that this is one of the most critical aspects of leadership and the overall accomplishment of the mission and success of the organization.

You can teach skills and processes; you can't teach passion.

One human being on fire for the mission can accomplish more than twenty who are there just for a paycheck."

As the Director of Operations and the CEO/Area Vice President of Operations for a healthcare organization, my direct reports included doctors, nurse practitioners, therapists, HR directors, and department directors.

I'm a very strong opponent of micro-managing. If you have to micro-manage a team member, you have the wrong person on the team. Micro-managing is a direct insult. I've discovered that micro-managers don't really know how to

"The steps of good men are directed by the Lord. He delights in each step they take."

Psalm 37:23 TLB

lead. They are busy asking you to report your minute-by-minute actions instead of being out in front like a true leader and delivering futuristic solutions and outcomes that will equip the team for success. The success of the mission is the goal, not monitoring movements.

> I've discovered extra blessings are found in the extra mile.

Hiring and promoting the wrong team members was one of the most potent lessons of my career. It was those I did the most for and helped the most who turned on me and did the most harm to me. Never expect too much from a human being.

It's extremely rare when loyalty isn't controlled by opportunity. Always remember, these same individuals will turn on anyone. They are only loyal to their boss at the time. This is where we learn to let go and trust God. Time has a way of revealing all things.

Permanent Solutions

I remember one of the first and greatest lessons I learned early in my leadership career. I was a supervisor for a Global Logistics Corporation. We had some vendors come out and make some repairs to the facility. The repairs weren't acceptable. I remember hearing our Director of Operations tell the man, "I need you to make permanent repairs." Those words have stuck with me forever. I do my best to apply them in all aspects of my life and leadership."

Permanent solutions are the target whether we are leading within the non-profit, ministry, or business sectors. Anything less is a waste of time and resources.

A perfect example of this is when I'm working with those in active addiction and alcoholism. They say, "I want to do "detox only," or I just need to attend the "outpatient program." My 20 years of experience have led me to the conclusion that these two decisions are equal to "putting a bandaid on the issue. They are short-term, temporary fixes.

When I meet people who are seeking a life free of drugs and alcohol, I always want them to experience true and lasting freedom. I know the permanent solution is a life powered by God's spirit. When we live according to His principles, we experience the best life any human will ever have.

In my life, Jesus is the permanent, eternal solution.

Chain of Command

Hidden agendas and much injustice thrive within the Chain of Command. Throughout my over two decades at all levels of leadership and multiple executive-level roles, I've experienced much. The Chain of Command only works when those reporting always tell the truth. When total honesty and integrity don't exist within the character of those doing the reporting, they are allowed to retaliate, bully, and block those they are jealous of and are trying to destroy secretly When those reporting are dishonest and have hidden agendas, they utilize their role as reporters to deliver injustice. They know those they dislike don't have a voice at the table. They know that if a team member reaches out to their boss, that team member will be retaliated against. It's a no-win situation for the individual who has done nothing to deserve what is taking place. Again, this is where the Kingdom Mindset is priceless.

When we witness God fight our battles repeatedly and witness His justice, we would have it no other way. The key is having the faith and patience to wait while God fights.

The Bait

Never let anyone trick you into aborting the mission God has given you to do. Our abilities and skill sets concerning responding and reacting will be the deciding factors that will determine whether we win or lose.

Remember, the offense is the enemy's bait to get you caught up.

When we fully understand that injustice is one of God's chosen methods of moving us to the next level, we understand, and it all makes sense.

If we take the bait, we get caught up in battles and chaos that we don't have to fight.

If we take the bait, we can lose access to those God has called us to reach with His love and healing. When we take the bait, the enemy can then discredit us.

Always remember telling the truth is not an emotional response.

The band Rage Against the Machine has a song entitled "Know Your Enemy."

Recognizing those the enemy sends to destroy you is key to winning the battle.

Not everyone whom you help, promote, or love is for you.

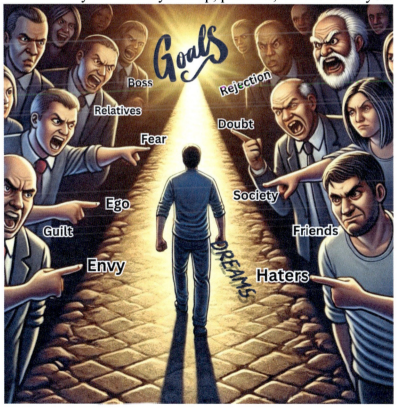

Many will smile, shake your hand, hug you, and then slice you apart behind your back. Do your best to protect yourself at all times.

Long Term Outcomes

In today's culture, we waste precious time if we aren't dealing with absolute truths and long-term outcomes. The data tells the story of what's real.

During my years as a leader, I've witnessed many initiatives and plans that look great initially, waste immense resources, money, and time, and never last. Most of what I've seen never last more than a few months. Again, this is when seeking permanent solutions, which is critical to long-term outcomes and success.

I've experienced many individuals and organizations seeking to take and make theirs any great new ideas. The critical issue here is that God gave the idea and vision to me and not them; God's favor will always accomplish more with less. I've discovered that stolen ideas rarely last. They always look great in the beginning. If you pay close attention, you will see they fade. The resources and teams slowly lose interest, and it's evident in the long run that God's favor is not there. I believe God intentionally and purposefully gives specific ideas, visions, and assignments to specific individuals.

Opposition

When operating in our culture today, we WILL face opposition. We will encounter people who come against us for no apparent reason.

God develops His strongest soldiers by giving them the most challenging and intense battles.

When we refuse to give up, we win. I've discovered that every time I experience injustice and opposition, I become stronger than before. How we emerge from the storm is proof of the wisdom we received as we endured.

When we fully understand that injustice and opposition are God's chosen methods to move us to the next level, we understand that God will make moves we would never make to get us to where He needs us to be.

What God has for us to do is of extreme importance. It is much more important than what we want or feel like doing. His plans and calling on our lives involve so many more people than just us, our immediate family, and our circle of friends.

The Power of Disqualification

Have you ever felt like God specifically develops and chooses the exact people who come against you? One of the greatest injustices I've ever experienced was when I was disqualified. I wasn't truly disqualified; I just thought I was.

A group of religious men, many of which were doing things and had done things I would not do, said I wasn't good enough to do things they were doing. They had found a single Bible verse that they learned how to use to discredit others, and at the same time, this verse was used to make them appear superior to others. I picture these men sitting around their family's dinner table, saying,

"Yeah, Stacy Dodd's not qualified to lead or perform weddings or funerals like we are. Another human being did something to him that he had no control over, and that disqualifies him. He's not spiritually and scripturally sound enough to do what we do."

Even though they had immense addictions to porn and flirted with many of the women in the Church being married, they were still superior. In their minds, they are spiritually superior. This makes them appear to be something they aren't in front of their wives and children.

It is amusing that they did and still do things I would never do. I often wonder how many men and women this group of men have done this to. I think of God sending people to His church to serve, and this group of religious men discourages and sends them away. I'll bet it's been hundreds. I've seen God's justice from time to time. I find comfort in knowing that their level of integrity is below what a leader in God's kingdom should be.

Since being "disqualified," God has publicly qualified me.

Remember, God doesn't call the qualified; He qualifies the called.

We become unstoppable when we allow injustices and opposition to fuel our fire and passion for the mission.

Since being "disqualified," God has blown my mind in how He's qualified me. I've had the honor and privilege of becoming an Ordained Minister. He gave me the most powerful ministry in the SE Region of the USA. My career with Bradford Health Services at Woodland Recovery Center has been ongoing, with multiple roles for almost ten years.

I've baptized over 800 men and women at the Recovery Center following the Sunday evening church services I lead weekly. I've led thousands to Christ in the DeSoto County Jail and at the Recovery Center. I've founded an award-winning youth mentorship program, shared my story hundreds of times, and even written four books. The entire region trusts me with their family members and loved ones to help them recover and find freedom from addiction and alcoholism.

From what I can tell, God chose me and ordained me. Despite this group of men deciding I wasn't as spiritual as they were, I've discovered that God does the calling and the qualifying.

Today, I'm very thankful for those men and what they did. The injustice fuels my passion for success.

Undercover Boss

If you've never watched the show "Undercover Boss," you should. This fantastic show features scenes when the CEOs and Founders of very successful organizations sneak undercover into their organizations to see what's happening.

Not only do they discover things that need to change, but they also get to meet and get up close and personal with the team members with the most incredible and touching personal lives and stories.

God is the ultimate "Undercover Boss." Never doubt that He knows all and sees all.

Our God knows everything about us. He's seen every tear. He knows the deepest desires of our hearts even better than we do.

God can give us our desires and secret petitions. The most amazing aspect of trusting in God's plan is that He protects us from ourselves as He gives us our desires. That's how He rolls.

I've never doubted God without having to apologize. Not even once!

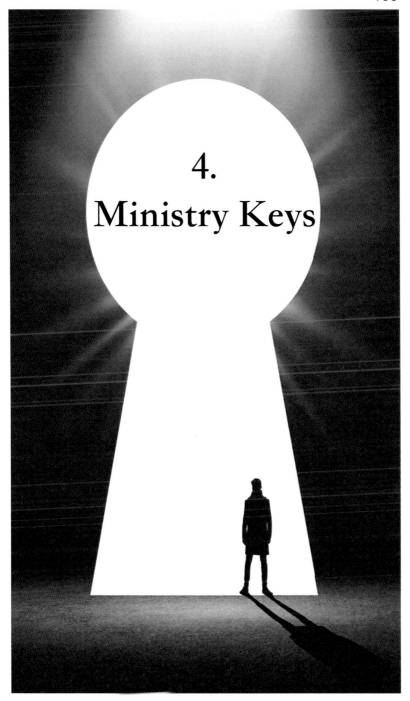

"I needed clothes and you clothed Me, I was sick and you looked after Me, I was in prison and you came to visit Me."

Then the righteous will answer Him, 'Lord, when did we see You hungry and feed You, or thirsty and give You something to drink?

When did we see you a stranger and invite You in, or needing clothes and clothe You? When did we see You sick or in prison and go to visit You?'

The King will reply, "Truly I tell you, whatever you did for one of the least of these brothers and sisters of mine, you did for Me."

Matthew 25:36-40 NIV

I always felt unworthy to serve God in any capacity, especially early in the transformation process. I remember like it was yesterday when I first started serving at Celebrate Recovery. My hands would tremble, my voice would quiver, and I would sweat when speaking to the group. It was horrible.

My Pastor, Denny Burt, never gave up on me. No matter how bad it got, He let me keep leading. This lesson he taught me by example has lived on in my heart and mind forever. Much like the lessons of unconditional love my mom and dad taught me, Pastor Denny's leadership and grace helped me keep going, even though my performance and thoughts would say otherwise. I pay this lesson forward every chance I get.

Another significant revelation I discovered concerning ministry is that, according to the truth and not religion, our past mistakes, shortcomings, pain, victories, and successes qualify us, not what some grandiose religious leaders in the Church use to disqualify us.

When I discovered the reasons God chose us, I was blown away. We connect with others through our weaknesses, not through our strengths. This means that my greatest strengths today are all of the bad decisions I made, the consequences I endured, the injustice I experienced, and the lessons I learned.

> "It's not about dying. It's about living for Jesus. Every day is the best day ever."
> *Aubrey Prigden, All Things New, Inc*

When I speak in recovery centers, schools, jails, and prisons across the USA, I'm extremely transparent and vulnerable. Sharing it all is a very humbling experience, but it can also set you truly and completely free from your past.

Celebrate Recovery

I began leading within the Global Christ-Centered Recovery Ministry of Celebrate Recovery in 2009. I had reached a point in my transformation and recovery where I was ready to give back.

When I think about my life today, I can't imagine how my life would've ended if I hadn't followed God's promptings to begin a life of service. Since that decision, I've been led to become Forever Friends with thousands of the most Beautifully Broken people in the Universe.

God intentionally used Celebrate Recovery to prepare me for what he had prepared for me. At Celebrate Recovery, I began leading Open Share Groups and Step Study Groups, sharing my testimony, and moved on to the role of Ministry Leader and Life Groups Director. I then became a Celebrate Recovery State Representative, and now Stephanie and I are Celebrate Recovery Inside State Representatives for North Mississippi and the Memphis Metro.

Celebrate Recovery Inside - Jails & Prisons

One of my favorite things to do is check into the jails and

prisons and share my story and my faith, which are the same. Access to those at Rock Bottom that God seeks is one of the greatest gifts a Christ-follower can ever ask for.

Knowing God's love is flowing directly through us into the hearts and minds of others is the supernatural experience of a lifetime. They are the TREASURE!

I work closely daily with the local Chaplains, Sheriffs, and Wardens to help those willing to get into programs. The majority I encounter in these facilities are struggling with childhood trauma and alcohol and drug addiction, which are, in fact, the same.

Due to God's direct leadership and our efforts in this wonderful ministry, we've witnessed thousands come to Christ and experience true freedom.

Mentorship

As the CEO and Founder of the Award Winning Youth Mentorship Program, The Hope Center, I'm engaged daily in our culture.

As a latch-key kid who grew up in the 1970s, I've experienced what can happen just hanging out in the neighborhood after school. That's where my drug and alcohol began.

In 2014, I received a call from one of my friends from Church. He said the DeSoto County Supervisors wanted to meet with us. When we met them, they asked us, "What can we do to help the City of Horn Lake?" There had been so many recent attacks by teenagers in Memphis that sparked unrest in our entire region. I asked them if we had a community center, and the answer was no. I've never understood why that wouldn't have been a priority long before I came along.

I had previously developed a for-profit business plan for an event center coffee shop. It was an incredible plan. However, I cared for my mom then, and I never really had the time to pursue this dream.

When I left the supervisor's office that day, God made it clear on my way home that I was to transform the for-profit business plan into a non-profit.

I scheduled an appointment with the Business College in Memphis and followed through with the plan's transformation.

Over the years, we have hosted many events in Horn Lake and throughout DeSoto County. Many key community leaders had the resources to help but have yet to do so.

I knew this calling was directly from God. So many times, I wanted to quit. I didn't have the money or energy to go on, and I didn't understand why the help wasn't there.

I remember one day standing at an event we planned at the Horn Lake Intermediate School. I stood by the front door, waiting for the kids to arrive. Only ten kids showed up that day, and my heart was broken. As tears rolled down my cheeks, I talked with God.

I never gave up on that dream. A lack of resources and

help forced me to get creative, and my passion intensified as God began to lead people to us. He led the exact people we needed.

One morning, while at work, I got a call. The operator said, "Retired Army Colonel Roy Ray is here to see you. I'm thinking,

"Why in the world would Roy Ray just show up at my office?"

He came in and sat down. He said,

"I'm with the Rotary, and we are looking for programs like yours to partner with. Would you like your program to become an official affiliate partner with the Memphis Grizzlies Foundation?"

Mr. Roy Ray was sent by God himself into our lives and the Hope Center mission. Since that day, the best executive-level leadership with MENTOR National has trained and equipped us. This is the elite mentoring organization in the USA.

Today, we mentor at-risk youth in DeSoto County, North Mississippi, and the Memphis Metro.

The Hope Community Center of North Mississippi is dedicated to empowering at-risk youth in 3rd to 12th grades. We create a safe and supportive environment to foster their growth and development, leveraging the national mentoring model of our partners in the Mentor Memphis Grizzlies Foundation to maximize our impact.

The Hope Center is a registered non-profit organization

with a 501(c)3 status. We have no building and no paid employees. We have been blessed to be invited into local schools and churches to be where the need is most prevalent. Our program is staffed by volunteers in the local community who have a passion for reaching the most vulnerable students.

All of our events are free to the students we serve. Our activities are sponsored through private and corporate donations. We are also an official Affiliate of the Mentor Memphis Grizzlies Foundation. Every dime we earn is used to bring activities, events, and materials to the youth in our community.

We focus on group mentoring and 1:1 mentoring of students in 3rd-12th grades. Growing up in today's world is challenging. Our mentoring team works with these students to give them a voice and help them as they mature into our future leaders. The benefits of mentorship are tremendous and much needed in today's climate and have been documented to reduce gang violence, increase leadership skills, reduce bullying, and increase school performance and citizenship.

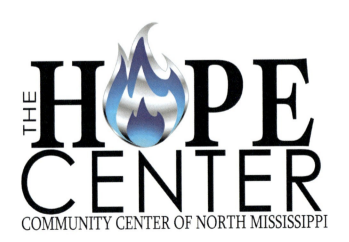

Jesus Christ is the ultimate leader and mentor. True mentorship replicates itself not by force but by example.

Jesus Christ never built a church building.

He built people.

He left us with 11 guys who changed history.

What are you leaving?

Not what …… but who?

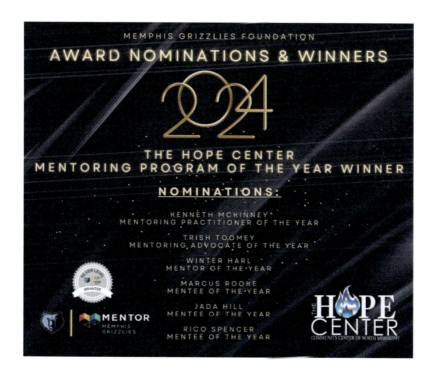

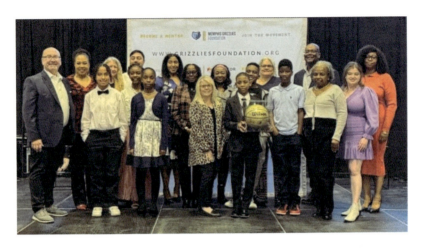

In 2023, The Hope Center advanced from Bronze to Silver Level Affiliate with the Memphis Grizzlies Foundation. We complete re-certification compliance reports annually and have developed an award-winning program.

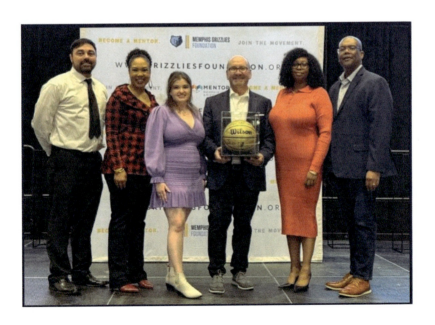

"Delight yourself also in the Lord, and He will give you the desires and secret petitions of your heart."

Psalm 37:4 Amplified

In 2023, I was nominated and selected to win the Mentoring Advocate of the Year from the Memphis Grizzlies Foundation.

In 2024, I was nominated and won the Non-Profit Leader of the Year from the Southaven Chamber of Commerce for my work with the Hope Center.

In 2024, The Hope Center was nominated and won the Mentoring Program of the Year award from the Memphis Grizzlies Foundation. We were selected from over 50 programs. I remember when I first started training in Memphis with top-level programs such as Streets Ministries, Youth Villages, and The Boys and Girls Club.

I always thought,

"I wish we could be at their level."

And guess what?

We won because we didn't give up and refused to quit, were humble enough to submit to authority, and were willing to see our resources as God's.

We won over all those programs I wished we could compete with long ago; in God's hands, dreams become realities.

Family

Growing up with a single mom, I became used to not having a typical family. My mom worked extremely hard and loved us unconditionally.

The holidays weren't what most families did.

On the other hand, my dad made sure his entire family was together at his home for Thanksgiving and Christmas. He didn't care who was mad at whom or who disapproved; he wanted us with him on the Holidays.

Family is very important to me today. I remember waking up one day, and I had lost it all. My family was tired and couldn't do it anymore. My addictions had worn us all out, including me. I would only go to family interactions as a way to maybe obtain a few bucks to continue my addiction. I was numb. The chemicals had stolen the love I had in my heart for others. At the end of my addiction, I would go weeks without encountering another human being. I was wandering around like a zombie lost on railroad tracks, through the woods, in abandoned houses, in and out of jail, humiliated and hopeless.

All that changed when I asked God to save and help me. The incredible thing is that He did. His spirit took up permanent residence within me, and He has been delivering on His promises ever since. My love for others and the fire within me only grow hotter and stronger by the day. I know who saved me and empowered me to live my life.

Having somewhere to go is home. Having someone to love is family. Having both is a blessing.

Today, I have a beautiful, funny, humble family that loves and laughs BIG.

My beautiful wife and best friend, Stephanie, is the solid rock that keeps us together. She always puts her family first and will fight anyone who messes with our family.

God has blessed me with a wonderful family. I had the honor of officiating at my step-daughter Kate and John's wedding and will soon officiate at my step-son Dustin and Amber's wedding.

I have three beautiful grandkids. They make me happy and give me a wonderful perspective. I'm blessed beyond measure.

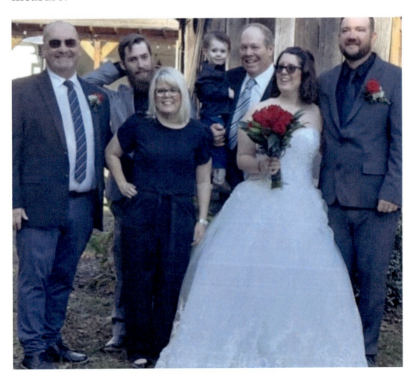

True Treasures

This life's "True Treasures" can't be purchased with money and power. The text messages I receive from those men and women God leads me to in the jails, prisons, recovery centers, hospitals, homeless shelters, and on Social Media are priceless. I print and frame these treasures.

Money can't buy a message in real life straight from the heart that was given freely. I've never prompted anyone to send me a message of gratitude or thanks.

God laid these treasures on their hearts and spoke to them clearly enough that they took action. They know how much I truly and genuinely care about them, and that means something to them.

When they spend time with me, leading the weekly Church services and Celebrate Recovery groups, they experience not only my words but also my actions. When they

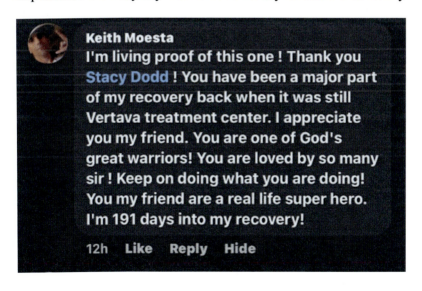

know I care enough to do more than just talk, they freely open up and show gratitude.

This is what sets people apart. It's the living proof of what's real and what's fake. Transparency and vulnerability open up the hearts and minds of those we're trying to reach.

This is a perfect example of FULL ACCESS to the Kingdom. God's spirit flows freely and unbridled through me, utilizing the access points and platforms to gain access to them. The activation of the Kingdom Keys, such as humility, transparency, and vulnerability, all work together perfectly to

> Stacy I finished your book and all I can say is WOW AWE Incredible. I had to stop several times as the Holy Spirt would overwhelm me. I'am 75 and have read hundreds or thousands of books but rarely have I finished them from cover to cover as I did yours.
> It has given me a NEW perspective and direction.
> I'll be ordering some to pass on in the Madison and Rankin jails hopefully next week.
> Moving forward in Christ Jesus.
> Thank you by brother.

access their hearts and minds.

When this magical and spiritual combination is put into action, actual transformations take place, and true and lasting freedom will be the long-term outcome.

> You have been SO right on everything youve said I would enjoy. Thank you Mr Stacy for the path you've shown me. I've never enjoyed sobriety and Jesus as much as i do at this moment. You really seem to get me and I trust you man. Thank you

I found these two gems when I was wandering the alleyways in Joplin when I was in the depths of my addiction. They are my most valuable treasure today. Their monetary value is very minimal. Their sentimental and spiritual value is

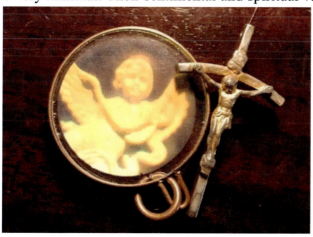

priceless.

They solidify that God was paying attention to every step I took. He knew then what would happen in my life after He took over. His plan is perfect. A God that sees past our current situation and junk into what we can become is mind-blowing. The fact that He can miraculously bring it all to pass is even more incredible.

I was handed This Book(Bible) in a very dark and lonely place. It's one of my prize possessions today. God knows exactly what we need, when we need it, and how to get it to us.

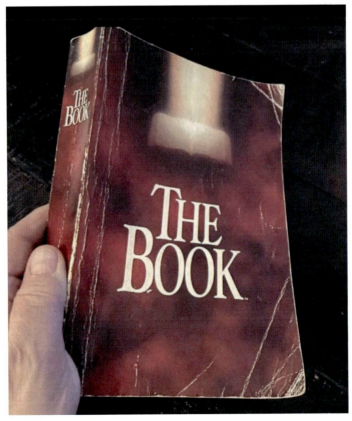

Missions

Missions have always fascinated me. I've studied mission work for quite some time now. I've discovered that people spend enormous amounts of time and resources on a picture.

When I think of missions, my first thoughts are about where the greatest need is.

I live in DeSoto County, a suburb of Memphis, Tennessee. Within a 20-mile radius of the community in which I live, we have the following on an immense, growing, unprecedented scale: Sex trafficking, assassinations, 12k untested rape kits, and more daily murders than all of the local news stations can report on, massive numbers of gang-related murders and crimes, record overdose incidents and deaths, immense teenage gang involvement, hunger, and the list goes on and on.

For the life of me, I will never understand why the majority of our local churches spend $10k to $30k on additional travel expenses to fly all around the world instead of helping our children, families, and communities right here at home. It doesn't make sense to me whatsoever.

I believe if every church in DeSoto County and the Memphis Metro would quit flying all over the globe with the giant teams and invest the same amount of time and resources here locally, our entire culture would be transformed. Just a thought!

Believe in You

One of the most complex struggles in my recovery journey was rebuilding my self-esteem. I had destroyed every drop I had. Only through my total dependence on God could I even begin the rebuilding process. It took years to build back. We must know that God honors His word, and we should never let anyone take that from us, regardless of our earthly title. Your past doesn't control God's will. When we belong to God and life comes against us for no reason, we must pay close attention and watch as He fights the battle for us. Self-esteem is so easy to lose and so hard to get back. Hold on to it with all you have. It belongs to you and no one else.

Always believe in yourself. Remember, the power of Christ living in you gives you the strength and energy to overcome all things. The Holy Spirit is key!

The Great Christian Cover-Up

I remember like it was yesterday when I surrendered my life to Christ. I discovered a new way of life. When I read the scriptures, I imagined a life in which people lived by the principles described in God's word. I assumed that all those who claimed their identity in Christ would live by His standards and teachings.

Boy, was I wrong. The more I got involved in the local church, the corporate world, and the business world, I found this couldn't be farther from the truth.

I discovered that identifying as a Christian was a "Great

Cover-Up." I found that people claim their identity in Christ and treat people horribly behind the scenes. I found that most arrogant and grandiose people claim their identity in Christ.

The main question I have is, how is it possible to publicly claim to love and honor Christ and expect His promises and protection, and to spend eternity with Him, and not live according to His standards?

I've discovered that claiming the identity of Christ is a great cover-up. Most people will never question a leader who claims to be a Christian loudly and publicly.

This and many other aspects is why it is what I call the "Great Christian Cover-Up."

Pastors & Politicians & Puppets & Worldly Titles

Some of the most extraordinary human beings I've ever met were Politicians. Some of the most deceitful human beings I've ever met were Politicians. Some of the most remarkable human beings I've ever met were Pastors. Some of the most deceitful human beings I've ever met were Pastors. I've met and been led by great CEOs. I've also met and been led by bad CEOs.

My first experience as God was teaching me the priceless gift and skill of discernment was when I was diagnosed with cancer in 2007.

I assumed that all doctors were good. I quickly found out that my assumptions were wrong, as they often are. My family and I were in the doctor's office in the exam room. The doctor came in and stated,

"You have bladder cancer."

And immediately left the room, went back into the hallway, and continued flirting with the nurses and laughing loudly. My family and I were in tears. I thought I was going to die. He failed to tell me it was treatable or anything to that effect. This experience was somewhat traumatizing. I changed doctors and had a wonderful experience. Today, I've been cancer-free for 17 years. There are wrong doctors. Lesson learned.

I've discovered visible and vast differences between Leaders and Politicians, as well as between Leaders and Pastors.

I've experienced and discovered that earthly and man-appointed titles no longer equal integrity. Only a human being's actions and example determine if they are a leader.

I believe that authentic, integrity-based leaders always do what's best for those they serve. It's never about control. It's always about the mission's success and taking ownership of the assignment and mission they are being paid to accomplish and trusted to do.

In my personal experiences, I've discovered that many Politicians, Pastors, and other top-level leaders operate within the Great Christian Cover-Up reality.

We have local politicians who pray for others loudly and publicly on social media, but behind the scenes, their lives don't match who they claim to be. The reality is that everyone knows the truth.

We have local Politicians and Pastors who demand total control of everything. If they can't have total control, they will miraculously come up with millions of dollars to build whatever organization suits their interests so they will have power. Instead of supporting organizations that are already effective and in place, they will spend millions of dollars that could've been utilized elsewhere to secure total control.

I've noticed they always find the money if it involves their personal interest, family, or especially their grandchildren. If it doesn't include them in these ways, they state, "We can't afford that.' We're being faithful stewards of the community's money." Once again, everyone knows. We watch huge facilities being built regularly, not for the community but for the politicians to have total control. It looks great for the next election, as well as the social media pictures and posts, but it's about so much more.

It's a huge disappointment, as I expected more from those trusted with more, especially those in higher positions who also claim their identity in Christ.

It's a double dose of lack of integrity.

Always base your view on the truth. Never assume that the title ensures integrity. Only the actual example and actions tell the story. Investigate thoroughly.

My lesson: Not everyone with the title of Pastor, Politician, CEO, Doctor, etc., is deserving.

Puppets is the term for those that Politicians and Pastors use to accomplish their control-based agendas. We have politicians who use local pastors to achieve their agendas. They privately fund the pastors and will do what they're told. They're being used. If they don't do what the Politicians say, they will never help them again.

One critical mindset that hurts the local church is the 'give me your money, work for free, and keep your mouth shut, or I (we) will never speak to you again' mindset, which is evident in most churches. You will discover this reality if you ever don't obey.

Leaders

I've worked closely with many types of leaders, as described below. We have the best leaders, the invisible leaders, and the cowardly leaders.

Experiencing the bad makes you appreciate the good so much more. The more time I spent around invisible and cowardly leaders, the more I witnessed firsthand what I never wanted to be, do, or be remembered as.

> "The first job of leadership is to love people. Leadership without love is manipulation." *Rick Warren, Pastor, Saddleback Church*

The Best

The best leaders are the ones you will never forget. These leaders don't view themselves as superior to those they lead or others who hold positions that they view as below them. They "always reply." The most outstanding leaders I've ever known had the busiest schedules and most responsibility. Guess what? They always took the time to reply to me. They knew it was a sign of respect. They also knew that they were in a leadership position to lead. That's what they are getting paid to do.

The best leaders are masters of validation, which is usually free. Refusing to validate is a direct sign of weak leadership arrogance and boasting. Leaders who refuse to validate only steal from themselves and the organizations and team members they lead.

The best leaders are always so far out in front of the team that they deliver futuristic solutions that drive the organization's long-term outcomes and will consistently outperform the competition. These leaders set the team up for success. It's intentional and precise.

The best leaders are brave leaders. They would never hide from those they serve. They wouldn't dare leave their team on the front lines to fight by themselves in the heat of the battle. They understand that when they are in the battle, it defines who they are. They don't hide in their offices and behind the lines. They are one with the team.

The best leaders operate from Integrity-based mindsets. When a leader doesn't always tell the truth, entire organizations, innocent families, and team members can be unjustly devastated. If dishonesty is a requirement to be at a top-level position and laughed about, this isn't integrity-based leadership.

The best leaders would never take credit for their team members' ideas and innovations. Over the years, I've shared many incredible ideas that have greatly impacted our organization. Only one time out of ten was I given credit. It's funny, as I was keeping track. The best leaders wouldn't dream of taking credit for their team's accomplishments. It's a sign of weakness and overall disrespect.

The best leaders don't act differently when their boss is in the room. They associate equally with all levels of the team. They don't worship their boss. When leaders act different when their boss is in town or the room, I promise the whole squad is sick to their stomach as they're forced to witness it. They notice. It's fake 100%.

Invisible Leaders

My first experience with invisible leaders taught me so much. When a leader is not onsite and directly involved with the day-to-day operations, many people will be forced to endure hardship and injustice. This is a result of only one person doing the reporting. They can cover up critical issues so they never get addressed. The entire organization can be in shambles, and the reporter can say, "Everything's just fine." The top-level leaders should visit and talk to everyone often. The only way trusting one will work is if that person is honest.

There is no middle ground with the truth.

Cowardly Leaders

The award-winning mentorship program I founded and currently lead focuses on bullying. Cowards and bullies do things to those who can't fight back. Professional bullies are cowardly leaders. They know that team members can't speak up even when telling the truth, as they know the bully will be allowed to retaliate and rearrange situations to terminate or eliminate that person. These leaders will take credit for their team's ideas and accomplishments, refuse to validate, and view themselves as much more important than the team. They block access to crucial individuals for those they are jealous of, minimize and/or ignore accomplishments, and maximize the struggles of those they seek to destroy.

I thank God every day that being led by cowardly leaders is a thing of my past today. I'm so glad I didn't give up when I endured these leaders. The only things that kept me going were that I knew God wanted me to have access to those struggling with active addiction, I had a responsibility to provide for my family, and I knew God's calling on my life was more important than my ego and pride. I wouldn't let weak, dishonest, arrogant, and grandiose individuals steal the blessings God has given and continues to give me.

The calling God has placed on my life is my responsibility. We must outsmart the enemy and strategically plan our responses. The Holy Spirit is the ultimate guide in the most intense battles.

The art of allowing God to fight our battles is a learned skill that demands patience, trust, and humility. His justice and final decisions are always worth the wait.

View From the Rocking Chair

"Be still and know that I am God."

Psalm 46:10

I decided long ago that I didn't want to reach the end of my life and wondered what could've happened if I had tried.

Today, I've learned to reach for the stars and pursue my hopes and dreams.

It's actually not for me. It's for those who may feel God's love flowing through me. It's for those families that have lost hope for their loved ones. It's for those in jail thinking life is over. It's for those kids who may choose a better life due to being involved in Hope Center.

When I get to the rocking chair, I won't have to think about what might have happened; I'm living what happened as I went for it and trusted God at His word!

I do it all out of immense gratitude for God reaching and saving me. It's the least I can do for this world for all God has given me.

Having FULL ACCESS to His Kingdom is the Greatest Gift of ALL!

THE END

Mr. Stacy Dodd is a NAADAC Nationally Certified Addiction Interventionist, Territory Manager for Bradford Health Services, Woodland Recovery Center, State Representative for the Global Christ-Centered Celebrate Recovery Inside Ministry, founder and CEO of The Hope Center of North Mississippi, and published author of four books.

He serves on the Board of Directors for the Southaven Chamber of Commerce, is an Ambassador to the Southaven Chamber of Commerce, and is an Ambassador to the Hernando Chamber of Commerce.

He travels daily throughout the SE Region of the USA. He utilizes his influence status on Social Media to identify and bring home any struggling with addiction and alcoholism.

As a public speaker, he travels to schools, jails, prisons, and recovery centers, speaks on addiction recovery, and shares his personal story.

He has built solid personal relationships with community leaders across North Mississippi and has spoken at statewide conferences on addiction and recovery.

Stacy Dodd is an author, speaker, and executive leader who overcame addiction to become a respected community and corporate leader.

His story starts with his book, "Backpack to the Burbs," and unfolds daily.

For speaking engagements, contact

stacydodd67@gmail.com.

stacydodd.com